Basic Concepts of Helping
A Holistic Approach

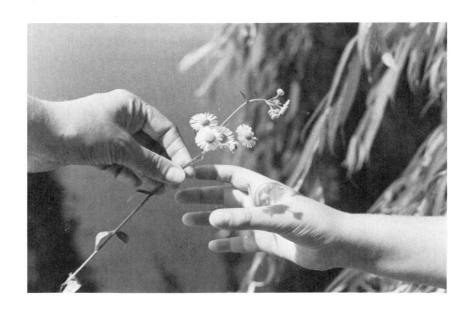

Photo credit to Mary Logan.

Second Edition

Basic Concepts of Helping
A Holistic Approach

Carolyn Cooper Hames, R.N., M.N.
Assistant Professor and Coordinator of
Parent–Child Health Nursing
College of Nursing
University of Rhode Island
Kingston, Rhode Island

Dayle Hunt Joseph, R.N., Ed.D.
Assistant Professor and Assistant Dean
College of Nursing
University of Rhode Island
Kingston, Rhode Island

APPLETON-CENTURY-CROFTS/Norwalk, Connecticut

0-8385-0559-7

Notice: The author(s) and publisher of this volume have taken care that the information and recommendations contained herein are accurate and compatible with the standards generally accepted at the time of publication.

Copyright © 1986 by Appleton-Century-Crofts
A Publishing Division of Prentice-Hall, Inc.

88 89 90 / 10 9 8 7 6 5 4 3 2

Prentice-Hall of Australia, Pty. Ltd., Sydney
Prentice-Hall Canada, Inc.
Prentice-Hall Hispanoamericana, S.A., Mexico
Prentice-Hall of India Private Limited, New Delhi
Prentice-Hall International (UK) Limited, London
Prentice-Hall of Japan, Inc., Tokyo
Prentice-Hall of Southeast Asia (Pte.) Ltd., Singapore
Whitehall Books Ltd., Wellington, New Zealand
Editora Prentice-Hall do Brasil Ltda., Rio de Janeiro

Library of Congress Cataloging in Publication Data

Hames, Carolyn Cooper, 1947–
   Basic concepts of helping.

   Includes bibliographies and index.
   1. Nurse and patient.   2. Helping behavior.
3. Holistic medicine. I. Joseph, Dayle Hunt, 1945–
II. Title. [DNLM: 1. Holistic Health—nurses' instruction.
2. Nurse–Patient Relations, WY 87 H215b]
RT86.H29 1986   610.73'069   85–13564
ISBN 0-8385-0559-7

Design: M. Chandler Martylewski

PRINTED IN THE UNITED STATES OF AMERICA

Dedicated to
Dr. Barbara Tate, who believed in us
and encouraged our professional growth
and to
Dr. Janet Hirsch, who with continued good humor and optimism,
has challenged our creativity

Contents

Preface

The second edition of *Basic Concepts of Helping: A Holistic Approach* continues to make a statement about the nature of helping and the importance of professional helpers. This book will acquaint students with the essential concepts that are a basis for professional helping. We believe there are certain attitudes, roles, and responsibilities that are germane to all helpers. Though written by nurses, this is a book that can easily be used by teachers, health care providers, clergy, social workers, and counselors.

Most beginning students bring little professional theory or experience with them to the classroom. Therefore, each new concept is explained first in terms of common every day life experiences and secondly in a professional context. Thus, the student can relate to and better understand the personal significance of a concept before he or she is expected to apply it in a professional setting. The term "client" has been chosen to refer to the person who is receiving assistance. We have tried to avoid the use of sexist phraseology.

This book is designed for students who are entering careers in helping. The concepts chosen are ones that we feel must be understood before engaging in the helping process. As in the first edition, the chapters are not placed in sequential order. Hence, the reader need not start with Chapter 1, "Adaptation." We encourage you to read those chapters that will best meet your needs. You may, for example, prefer to start with the concept of group (Chapter 3) if you are in a classroom setting.

Appendix I consists of a collection of games and activities that have been successfully used by us in our teaching. Not only are they fun, they emphasize major concepts, enhance empathy, and stimulate group discussion. Many of our most effective techniques, however, are simple, spontaneous ideas that seemed appropriate for a particular class. We encourage you to use these activities as presented or adapt them as you like.

The idea for this book originally emerged from an undergraduate course taught at the University of Rhode Island. Students from a variety of colleges take the course and laud its relevance to their career choice. They frequently tell us that this book "grows" with them. As they become more professionally knowledgeable and experience more complex situations with clients, they increasingly recognize the importance of having a firm foundation in the basic concepts of helping. We hope that you, too, will reread the book from time to time.

Acknowledgments

As in any venture of this magnitude, we are indebted to some special people. A sincere thanks to our colleagues who shared and constructively criticized so well; to Elizabeth Diaz and David Warren, students who brilliantly reviewed the chapters; and our editors, Charles Bollinger and Susan Neitlich, at Appleton-Century-Crofts, who have encouraged us through the writing of two editions. We wish to give special acknowledgment to Marylee Evans, Brenda Bissell, and Jane Fanning for their contributions of chapters in the first edition. We would like to thank our families for their loving support and encouragement throughout this project. Last, but not least, our grateful appreciation is extended to Joyce Deacon for her flawless typing and to Peggy Haggerty for her ability to capture the essence of helping on film.

Basic Concepts of Helping

of Helping

A Holistic Approach

Life belongs to the living, and he who lives must be prepared for changes.
Johann Wolfgang von Goethe

1

Adaptation

Upon completion of the following reading and suggested exercises, the student will be able to:
1. Discuss a personal philosophy of life.
2. Define the purpose of a theoretical framework.
3. Describe the usefulness of theory when helping clients.
4. Describe how adaptation theory integrates the biophysical, psychosocial, and cognitive components of the person.
5. Define the nine characteristics of adaptation.

This is a book about helping people. Its main thrust is to provide the novice helper with information that is germane to all helping encounters. The concepts and principles of helping are broad and, therefore, applicable to all professional helping situations. Those of you who are contemplating a career in nursing, teaching, counseling, medicine, physical or occupational therapy, social work, dentistry, pharmacy, etc., will find that the concepts presented in each chapter relate to your chosen profession. It is the authors' intent to enrich your knowledge, to share some simple communication skills, and to encourage you to analyze critically your approach to people.

Helping is a far more difficult process than first perceived by the new helper. Liking people and wanting to assist them are necessary qualities, but they alone are not sufficient to fulfill the comprehensive task of professionally

1

helping. It is fundamental that you study both the art and science of being a skilled, responsible professional helper.

THE SELF

One of the first steps in becoming an effective professional helper is to learn more about yourself. "The self is the center of a person's existence, his frame of reference for dealing with life" (Combs, 1973, p. 144). As you develop insight into yourself as a person, you will find it easier to relate to others. You will become cognizant that each of us is an individual with unique ideas about life and how to cope with its problems.

The self-concept develops gradually from infancy through adulthood. It evolves as a result of interactions with parents, peers, siblings, and the general sociocultural milieu (Gale, 1969). As you enter the helping relationship, you bring with you perceptions of yourself and how you interact with people. Your self-concept is quite complex in nature. It is the result or product of your physical, emotional, moral, ethical, and intellectual development. The stronger and more accurate your self-concept, the easier it will be for you to help others. Research findings indicate that people with high self-concepts have more confidence in themselves (Fitts, 1965).

The self-concept is not fixed—it is forever changing. Hence, it is important that you "get in touch" with your feelings and insecurities in an attempt to positively strengthen your self-concept. Before you can help others, you must first develop a "firm foundation from which to deal with the problems of life" (Combs, 1973, p. 145). You must learn who you are. You must know your strengths as well as your weaknesses. You must gain an awareness of when you are independently capable and when you need to rely on others.

As you read the chapters in this text, it is imperative that you closely examine your own reactions to the concepts discussed. Each of you will read this book from a slightly different perspective, depending upon your life experiences thus far. You may note when reading the chapter on culture, for example, that your knowledge about the customs and mores of others is limited. This is an opportunity to begin learning about people who are different from you. As your knowledge about the complexity of professional helping increases, you will see how important it is to understand your own self and to be accepting of others. React as honestly as possible to the exercises and the tasks asked of you in this text. Do not be afraid to admit your biases or shortcomings. We all have them! It is your insight into them that helps you to grow and change.

PHILOSOPHY

As you begin to examine who you are and what you believe, you will begin to identify some of your biases. Your basic value system, like your self-concept, has evolved as you have matured. Your philosophical beliefs reflect many aspects of your life. These beliefs have been reflected by your interpersonal relationships, religion, education, social status, and so on. You may, in fact, find that some of your values will change over time; the intent of this text, however, is to have you reexamine rather than change your value system. Insight into who you are and how your beliefs and background influence your approach to people will be extremely helpful in the interactions that you will eventually have with clients. Your philosophy will affect the way you perceive people and events and, therefore, will influence the way you respond to them.

Do you believe, for instance, that all people are basically good and do the best they can given their circumstances? Or do you think some people are inherently evil and freely hurt and abuse others for their own gain? Common sense suggests that as a professional helper your intervention with clients will be affected by your beliefs about human nature. You also must begin to recognize that your own notions of right and wrong—whether they are related to moral, legal, spiritual, ethical, educational, or health issues—must be carefully monitored so you will avoid a judgmental attitude when helping others.

It is important to realize that people are not always able to articulate their philosophies. More commonly, they simply act them out. Most of us, however, have strong beliefs about why we live our lives as we do. Look at the following example, using the issue of cigarette smoking:

> Harry, aged 49, continues to smoke one pack of cigarettes per day. He argues that life is a gamble and death is inevitable. He has decided to enjoy as many "pleasures" as he can find. Chet, aged 45, has not smoked for 10 years. He cites research findings that smoking causes heart and lung disease. Chet prefers to relinquish some of life's pleasures to enable him to live a healthier life.

Here are two opposing viewpoints, each having a reasonable rationale. There exist very radical differences in Harry's and Chet's philosophical beliefs about life. Helpers must recognize these differences and prudently avoid imposing their own philosophical beliefs upon clients.

Because one's philosophy changes with time and circumstance, it is important for professional helpers to continually reexamine their beliefs and attitudes about people. "Individuals use their philosophy of life, to orient themselves to the world around them" (Flynn & Heffron, 1984, p. 4). Hence, an understanding of your own philosophy can assist you when helping others. You are not going to be asked to relinquish your own beliefs, but rather you are asked to appreciate and respect that philosophical differences exist among people.

THEORETICAL FRAMEWORKS

As you begin to examine your attitudes and beliefs about the nature of the person, you also must determine appropriate approaches to helping. During your professional education you will learn many new facts, theories, concepts, and skills pertinent to your career choice. You will need to organize them in some systematic, meaningful way. Theoretical frameworks help you to do this. Theoretical frameworks—or conceptual models, as they are sometimes called—lend structure to a situation and, therefore, enhance problem solving. Consider the following:

> The Walshes have always approached parenthood with certain expectations of their children. In an effort to foster their growth into mature adults, the Walshes have always maintained that the children must be responsible for certain household chores. Thus, David, who is 15, is expected to straighten his room, clean up after the evening meal, and prepare his 4-year-old brother, Johnathan, for bed. The Walshes believe that children are part of the family group and, therefore, should share in some of the routine household chores.
>
> David has been handling these responsibilities since he was 13 years old. He enjoys his time with his younger brother, Johnathan, and appreciates the fact that his parents need some time to rest after the evening meal. However, his sophomore year in high school has become quite demanding—he is in honors courses, on the yearbook staff, and on the football team. He is beginning to feel overwhelmed. It is usually eight o'clock before he can begin studying, and sometimes he does not have enough time to finish all his work.
>
> His parents have always been faithful to a parenting framework that encourages participation of children. Their basic philosophy stems from the belief that responsible children grow into responsible adults. However, they are beginning to question the amount of responsibility David is handling. They decide that at present he needs to be responsible for his student role and, therefore, should be relieved of some of his household chores. His parents have not changed their beliefs about childrearing; they have just changed the mechanism by which David learns about responsibility, i.e., school activities rather than home activities.

In professional helping situations the theoretical framework enhances client assessment and the development of appropriate interventions. The theoretical framework provides the guidelines for caring, while the philosophy provides the helper with a value system for prioritizing care (Bevis, 1982). It is most important, however, that the theoretical framework selected by a professional be congruent with the professional's basic philosophical beliefs, since the framework will provide direction to the professional's approach to helping.

For example, a Freudian psychoanalyst views the client from an entirely different perspective than does the behavioral psychiatrist. Neither approach is more correct than the other; they differ simply by directing the helpers toward assessment of different kinds of information from the client. The Freudian psychoanalyst will design interventions appropriate to that framework. The behavioral psychiatrist will probably choose interventions slanted toward his or her framework.

A conceptual model also must be useful for the client as well as useful and compatible to the helper. It addresses the needs of both. If appropriately selected, the theoretical framework allows the helper to respond to the client in a creative fashion and to consider the client's total personality. If a theoretical framework is utilized to gather information about a client, that assessment will be comprehensive and wholistic. Thus, selection of a theoretical framework that is consistent with one's philosophy and appropriate for assessment of one's client population is essential for responsible professional practice.

THEORY—ITS RELATIONSHIP TO HELPING

The term *theory* is probably familiar to you. "Like most terms, theory has multiple meanings" (Chinn & Jacobs, 1983, p. 2). You have all heard the term theory used to express an idea of why something has happened. Note the following example:

> Peggy and Anita are 23-year-old housemates presently discussing their roommate Joan's apparent difficulty relating to men.
>
> *Peggy:* My theory is that Joan is so eager to please that she scares her dates away.
>
> *Anita:* You know—now that you mention it, I think you are right.
>
> *Peggy:* She's always available—she doesn't seem to know when to say no.

In this example Peggy has a theory or an idea about why Joan has trouble relating to men.

Obviously, theory is not quite as simplistic as the example leads you to believe. Although theory is based upon ideas and hunches, it also involves rigorous methods of systematizing information.

The purpose of theory is to guide the helper in understanding human nature. Theory is an abstract "representation of reality; it is not reality itself" (Chinn & Jacobs, 1983, p. 3). Theory is useful in that it depicts events or aspects that are essential for understanding the client's world. Stevens (1984, p. 1) compares theory to a map "which picks out those parts that are important for a given purpose." Hence, the use of theory assists the helper in identifying the important stimuli that influence the client's response to life.

Theories allow us to describe and explain why something has happened and eventually to predict what will happen (Kim, 1983). You began learning about theory in elementary school when you studied such famous people as Copernicus and his beliefs about why the earth revolves around the sun. Throughout your education you have been acquainted with various theories. Some have proved to be most useful. For example, scientists learned long ago that giving a person small doses of the bacterium causing a particular disease actually prevents the person from developing that disease. As a result, smallpox has been eradicated.

Other theories have proved to be erroneous. For example, Ptolemy's theory, which stated that the earth was stationary and at the center of the universe, influenced the thinking of scientists for nearly a thousand years.

Like scientists, professional helpers base their practice on theory. While this may not have always been the case, we have become quite sophisticated and scientific in our approach to caring. We have adopted much of what we know from the social and physical sciences. Some of our theory is still developing. One thing is clear, however: in this decade it is ludicrous to approach helping relationships as trial-and-error experiences. "Theory is an intellectual tool used to explain the world in which we live" (Kim, 1983, p. 10). It is at times complex and obtuse, yet it guides our care and gives credence to our practice.

Thus, we see that professional helpers have some degree of choice in directing their practice. Once they have learned the facts, concepts, and theories appropriate to their profession, they select those most consistent with their philosophy and most effective for their particular clients. Clearly, a great deal of responsibility and accountability is expected and assumed.

ADAPTATION

The concept of adaptation has been shown to be useful for professional helpers. Harry Helson (1964) originally proposed the adaptation-level theory, and since then others such as Roy (1970, 1971, 1973, 1980) have altered Helson's basic concepts so that his ideas are more readily applicable to helping clients in a health care setting. Adaptation has been so popular among health care providers that it is frequently selected—in its broadest sense—as a theoretical framework. Such is the case for this text.

One of the most important assumptions of adaptation theory relates to the proposition that people respond to their environment in totality. The environment consists of three domains or modes. These modes are similar for all people and are useful to helpers in various social science disciplines. The use of modes or domains helps to organize information about a person schematically and then to transcend that information by unifying the domains and examining the person as a whole.

Adaptation theory posits that three modes—biophysical, psychosocial, and cognitive—must be carefully examined before helpers can decide upon a plan of action. The person cannot respond in a solitary mode. Adaptation in one mode necessitates alterations, however minute, in the other two modes. Hence, the modes overlap and interrelate. Figure 1–1 depicts the overlapping modes.

The Adaptation Modes

The biophysical mode concerns itself with the person's physical and genetic makeup. The emphasis in this mode is on the body and how it functions. It

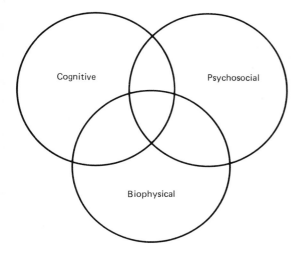

Figure 1-1. The interrelationships of the three modes: the totality of the person.

is believed that stimuli from the internal and external environment impinge upon the person and cause a biophysical response (Hames, 1978). Certainly, biophysical alterations are important, and their input must not be underestimated. However, people are more than biophysical beings, and we must remember that what occurs at a cellular level is only a portion of the adaptation process. The helper who feels that this mode alone is important denies the client his or her inalienable right to holistic care—to be viewed as a whole person.

The psychosocial mode concerns itself with the client's psychological, sociological, and spiritual self. It is believed that certain stimuli impinge upon the behavior pattern or coping mechanism that the individual normally uses in adjusting to people, society, and culture (Hames, 1978). This mode, perhaps more than the other two modes, attests to individual differences and the uniqueness of clients. Understanding the client's psychosocial response is not an easy task; it takes time to come to know the person.

The cognitive mode concerns itself with the client's ability to understand what is occurring in his or her world. This mode examines stimuli that influence the client's use of learning, perception, reasoning, and communication (Hames, 1978). Without a careful assessment of this mode, the possibility of effective client teaching is markedly diminished.

It should be emphasized that categorization of the individual into three modes merely facilitates assessment. Ultimately, the modes interconnect to become whole or, as some may argue, greater than whole.

> The whole is always greater than the sum of its parts. In other words, each part standing by itself has a certain meaning or value that is enhanced or altered, i.e., it becomes "greater", when it is in interaction with the other system elements. (Heffron, 1984, p. 12)

Consider the patient who has been diagnosed as having a terminal disease. Merely to investigate the disease and its effects upon the person's body only tells part of the story. Once it is learned that the client is deeply religious, believing in a life hereafter, our plan of care, our psychological support, will be much more pertinent to the patient's real needs.

One might argue that helpers from some professions do not need to examine all three modes closely. The following examples illustrate that only with three-mode assessment can holistic care be given.

> Think about the local pharmacist who fills Mr. Hart's prescription monthly. Clearly, it is important that the pharmacist be cognizant of the action and effect of medication on the body. Think, however, about this type of information coupled with the pharmacist's assessment of the client's ability to self-medicate and to recognize untoward side effects from the drug. Certainly, the knowledge gained when examining each mode enhances the kind of care delivered to the client.
>
> Consider the priest who encourages his parishioner, Mr. Ellis, to become involved with the church's music program. The priest recognizes that the parishioner is a skilled musician who will personally gain psychologically and cognitively from this participation. He knows further that Mr. Ellis has a past history of illness and, though the priest's profession is not biophysically oriented, he cautions the client about overextending himself.

The Nature of Stimuli

It will be evident from the discussion that follows that adaptation theory is based upon a stimulus–response model. In other words, all of a person's behavior is caused by a stimulus. This stimulus induces a response, which, in turn, causes a behavior.

$$\text{Stimulus(i)} \rightarrow \text{Response(s)} \rightarrow \text{Behavior(s)}$$

As in most theoretical frameworks, there is some new terminology for you to learn. It will be easier for you to understand the theory if you make an effort to learn these terms. Helson (1964) is credited with identifying three categories of stimuli that bombard the person continually throughout life. Stimuli are defined as the internal or external forces that cause, or have a tendency to cause, some directional change in an individual's life (Helson, 1964).

There are three particular kinds of stimuli that influence people. The strongest stimulus is the *focal stimulus*. This stimulus presents itself most immediately to a person. For example, if the client is having a tooth drilled at the dentist and refuses Novocain, it is likely that the drilling of the tooth is the focal stimulus during that period of time. It is important to remember that there is only one focal stimulus presenting itself at a given moment in time. Furthermore, that focal stimulus must be examined in each of the three modes—biophysical, psychosocial, and cognitive—for a thorough assessment of the client's behavior. Thus, in the biophysical mode, the person may have pain as a result of the drilling. In the psychosocial mode, the drilling may elicit a stoic response and the client may state, "I can tolerate this." In the cognitive mode, the drilling may elicit knowledge that the pain is only temporary. The patient realizes that in 20 minutes it will all be over.

Identifying the focal stimulus is not an easy task, as it can change from moment to moment. Thus, the drilling of the tooth may be the focal stimulus for only part of the visit. As the dentist begins to fill the tooth, the suction apparatus causing dryness in the mouth may become the focal stimulus for that moment in time.

To discuss the client's world as merely a result of a focal stimulus would be shortsighted. Clients do not live in vacuums. They are continually being bombarded by all sorts of internal and external stimuli, and this combination of stimuli dramatically affects their response to the environment.

Contextual stimuli are always present in conjunction with the focal stimulus. Contextual or background stimuli are those forces exerting an influence upon the person's behavior at the same time as the focal stimulus. They originate in either the internal or the external environment. Hence, the noise of the drill, the awkward position of holding the mouth wide open, the soothing music in the dentist's office, the skilled manual dexterity of the dentist, and an understanding of what is being done all act to influence the client's response to this particular dental visit. There are usually several contextual stimuli in the biophysical, psychosocial, and cognitive modes that influence the client. Unlike the focal stimulus, contextual stimuli can remain the same or vary from mode to mode. The noise of the drill and the awkward mouth position can be classified as biophysical stimuli because they directly involve physical aspects of the body. The soothing music and the skilled manual dexterity of the dentist can be classified as psychosocial in nature because they provide a calming influence and a degree of confidence. Certainly, if the client has been told what to expect, he or she knows something about what is happening; hence, this contextual stimulus would be classified in the cognitive mode.

Since adaptation theory allows for fluidity, it must be understood that the focal stimulus does continually change. A contextual stimulus can, at a given moment, become the strongest stimulus and, therefore, be the new focal stimulus. It also must be remembered that people are bombarded with many contextual stimuli at one time. In reality, it may not be practical or feasible to study all of these stimuli. It is important for the helper to learn how to prioritize these stimuli and to recognize which of them are more potent in influencing the client's behavior. In the particular case of the dentist's office, the manual dexterity of the dentist and the awkward position of the mouth are probably of high intensity and, therefore, quite influential in the client's response to this situation.

Residual stimuli are those forces stemming from the person's cultural and genetic background. Residual stimuli reflect the client's value system and his or her past experiences in life. These stimuli are often difficult to identify, since the helper may not really know much about the client's past. Residual stimuli are one of the reasons why perceptive, accurate history taking is so important in many helping professions. In the above example, the hereditary nature of dental caries definitely influences the genetic condition of teeth and, thus, lends itself nicely to a biophysical classification. The fact that the client has been told from childhood that having teeth filled is a painful process influences his or her psychosocial response. The client's knowledge about dental caries and their deleterious effect influences the cognitive response.

Helpers are expected to identify each of these three categories of stimuli and to determine how they influence the client's behavior. In this particular example, that behavior could range from straining to keep the mouth open to remaining silent, wincing, or screaming. It is important that the helper in this case, the dentist, be cognizant of those behaviors. If the dentist recognizes these behaviors, the approach to care will be altered—something will be done to make the client more comfortable.

A word of caution must be exercised at this point. The foregoing discussion attests to the mechanics of how one theory can be put into practice by the helper's using a theoretical framework. Theory, however, is a dynamic process that helps us to understand the holistic nature of the person. Adaptation is a holistic theory that allows its users to identify the interrelatedness of component parts in the whole system (Heffron, 1984). The three modes are not examined independently; the ultimate aim of the theory is to unify the modes in an attempt to understand each individual's uniqueness in relationship to the experiences he or she encounters. Humans are complex beings, and the adaptation framework suggested in this text encourages examination of this complexity.

Meaning of Adaptation

The term *adaptation* has several meanings, depending upon the particular discipline being studied. The anthropologist thinks of adaptation as evolution of a culture in an attempt to meet changing environmental demands. The biologist thinks of adaptation as a process to restore homeostasis within the person's internal environment. The psychologist thinks of adaptation as a process that helps individuals to cope emotionally with their environment (Phipps, Long, & Woods, 1983). Many other professional helpers have an even broader perspective of adaptation in that they believe it is a process by which the client copes with changes in his or her internal and external environment (Rambo, 1984).

Adaptation is a process by which people change in response to stimuli within their internal and external environment. If adaptation is successful, the person's balance is not disturbed. "If the adaptation is faulty, the person becomes ill and as a sick person he must adapt to illness" (Luckmann & Sorenson, 1974, p. 11). Adaptation is an ongoing process that occurs throughout life. Human adaptation is complex and inclusive of the biophysical, psychological, and cognitive modes. If the person is successful in coping with life's stresses, the adaptation is considered high level or positive in nature. However, if the person is unable to withstand life's stresses and subsequent coping mechanisms falter, the adaptation is at a low level or is negative in nature.

"Adaptation is a constant, ongoing process that occurs along the time continuum, beginning with birth and ending with death" (Brunner & Suddarth, 1984, p. 121). Unlike many contemporary theorists, the followers of adaptation theory refute the notion of maladaptation. This theory postulates that the person who is alive continually interacts with the environment and adapts accordingly. Adaptive behavior is referred to as ranging from high to low levels. The mere fact that the person is living attests to the fact that he or she is adapting, although the strength of his or her adaptive mechanisms may be so poor that a high quality of life cannot be sustained. The term maladaptation is equated with death, meaning that the person who has died is no longer capable of adapting to the environment.

When assessing the person's level of adaptation, the helper must carefully consider the value system of the client. Judgments about the client must be made from the client's reference system, rather than the helper's. It is not unusual for the helper to note a conflict between personal value systems and those of the client. Disregarding the client's values not only does the person a disservice, but enhances a lower rather than a higher level of adaptation. Note the following example:

> Maisy is a 35-year-old woman who lives in a five-room tenement house with her eight children. Her husband works as a laborer but is often out of work because of a back injury. You are presently talking with Maisy in the gynecology clinic. She has just miscarried her ninth child. As you enter the room, she is sobbing and saying, "I'm so disappointed. This was a real special baby. What if it is my last pregnancy?"

What is your initial reaction to Maisy's question? Can you appreciate her feelings? Do you think she should be relieved about the miscarriage? Have you ever thought about children bringing wealth to a culture? Can you recognize how your value system might influence Maisy's adaptation level?

Earlier in this chapter the point was made that philosophical beliefs should be congruent with theoretical beliefs. Helpers must be careful not to impose their philosophical beliefs on the client. Helpers must further ensure that the theoretical framework they use when assessing clients encourages value-free judgments.

Characteristics of Adaptation

Beland and Passos (1981), Brunner and Suddarth (1984), Luckmann and Sorenson (1974), Rambo (1984), and others have identified several characteristics that are pertinent to this discussion of adaptation and to your conceptualization of the client as a person. They are as follows:

1. *Adaptation involves the entire organism.* The person always responds to the environment in a holistic manner. Think of the 40-year-old mother of two teenage children who learns that her husband has just died unexpectedly. Her response will be quite complex. You would expect that she will cry and talk about what life will be like without her husband (psychosocial). She may further begin to arrange the funeral plans according to what she feels her husband would want (cognitive). She may have difficulty sleeping and have a loss of appetite (biophysical). Regardless of the particular behaviors, it is apparent that a total response occurs. Although each mode could be studied independently, in reality they are interwoven to produce a functioning person with inseparable biophysical, psychosocial, and cognitive needs (Rambo, 1984).

2. *The person is in constant interaction with a changing environment.* The individual is continually bombarded with internal and external stimuli. For example, consider how each of you interacts daily with changing weather conditions. These conditions often influence how we respond to daily activities. Probably all of you have suffered from occasional attacks of "spring fever" or "rainy day blues."

3. *Adaptive mechanisms within the body always attempt to maintain homeostatic conditions.* Within the person's body there exist certain safeguards that protect the person from injury. When a bone is fractured, for example, the body's response is to develop procallus. This procallus formation is simply an "overgrowth" of bone, and its function is to splint the broken bone fragments, protecting the bone from further injury.

4. *The organism usually uses an adaptive response that is economical.* The previous example demonstrates the way the body responds to healing and prevents deformity. Procallus formation is also economical because in its absence the bone fragments would be more difficult to align and thus take longer to heal.

5. *Adaptation is a dynamic process involving active participation from the person.* The person is usually aware of stressors in the environment and is able to take some type of preventive action. For example, whenever John Doe is confronted with overwhelming stimuli, he is able to release some of his tension by laughing, crying, or fighting. Remember studying for a big exam—feeling very pressured about getting a good grade? Some of you were able to spend hours studying with little rest.

6. *Psychological adaptations are more numerous than biophysical adaptations.* It is understandable that within the body there exist narrow limitations within which life can continue. Hence, when blood sugar exceeds a certain level, death may occur if the basic underlying condition is untreated. Choices for adapting in an emotional sense are considerably more numerous because in the psychological realm there usually does not exist this "fine line" between life and death.

7. *It is more difficult for the client to adjust to sudden rather than pro-longed changes in adaptation.* The period of time involved in making an adjust-ment is crucial to the client's ability to respond appropriately. Think for a moment of the mother who has learned that her child has been killed in an automobile accident. Would this same mother react differently to the death of a child who has had leukemia for many years?

8. *There are limits to the process of adaptation.* The inherent ability to adapt is related to the person's genetic and emotional makeup. Thus, a person with limited intellectual ability would not be successful in a curriculum de-signed for students with average capabilities. The patient who suffers from congestive heart changes is limited as to the amounts and type of activity that can be tolerated.

9. *The ability to adapt varies from person to person.* "A . . . feature of adaptation is that the more flexible the organism in its capacity to adapt, the greater the capacity to survive" (Beland & Passos, 1981, p. 75). To illustrate this concept:

> Christin and Kara are both married students enrolled in the College of Pharmacy. Christin constantly complains about all the work she has to do at home and in school. She is "getting by," but spends most of her time lamenting unhappily her plight in life. Kara is easygoing, laughs a lot, and does well in school. She enjoys getting involved in extracurricular activities and is actively involved with her son's hockey team.

"Flexible individuals who are readily responsive to change, and who employ a wide range of compensatory mechanisms, are more adaptable than those persons lacking these qualities" (Luckmann & Sorenson, 1974, p. 15). Consequently, those people who are able to adapt at a high level to the vary-ing stimuli of life are usually better able to withstand stress than people who are rigid.

Adaptation—A Holistic Approach

In this discussion of adaptation, the emphasis has been placed upon the per-son's ability to adapt holistically—biophysically, psychosocially, and cognitively. For some of you, this apparent dissection of the person into three compartmental categories means stripping the person of his or her uniqueness—of his or her wholeness. The intention of this chapter is, in fact, the opposite. Its purpose is to demonstrate how the three modes unite and over-lap, thus making the client a whole rather than a fragmented person.

The body and the mind are not two separate entities. One influences the other and if the body or the mind fails, the person's adaptation to life is in-complete. If both body and mind fail us, our ability to adapt may be lost, and death may ensue.

"Man's ability to respond positively, or to adapt, depends upon the degree of change taking place and the state of the person coping with the change" (Roy, 1976, p. 12). Therefore, the way in which people adapt to their environment depends upon the number and intensity of stimuli influencing them, their response to these stimuli, and their personal resources (mind and body.)

A FINAL NOTE

The intent of this chapter is to acquaint the helper with the importance of philosophy and the purposes of theory, and to present an example of a framework—adaptation—that can easily be applied to any number of helping disciplines. As you continue with your education, you will be introduced to a variety of theories and frameworks. In time you will probably come to embrace that which works best for you. This framework should help you to examine the client in a systematic fashion and to consider the client's needs from a holistic perspective. Theory should always guide your practice; it is the cornerstone of all helping professions.

IMPORTANT REMINDERS

1. The theoretical framework selected by a professional should be congruent with the professional's basic philosophical beliefs.
2. Theory guides helpers in their search for an understanding of human nature.
3. Adaptation theory encourages viewing the client in a holistic fashion.
4. According to adaptation theory, the client's environment consists of three modes: biophysical, psychosocial, and cognitive.
5. Theory is dynamic in nature; its purpose is to focus on important events that influence the client's response to life.

REFERENCES

Beland, I., & Passos, J. (1981). *Clinical nursing. Pathophysiological and psychosocial approaches* (4th ed.). New York: Macmillan.

Bevis, O. (1982). *Curriculum building in nursing—A process* (3rd ed.). St. Louis: C. V. Mosby.

Brunner, L., & Suddarth, D. (1984). *Textbook of medical-surgical nursing* (5th ed.). Philadelphia: Lippincott.

Chinn, P. L., & Jacobs, M. K. (1983). *Theory and nursing—A systematic approach.* St. Louis: C. V. Mosby.

Combs, A. (1973). *Helping relationships.* Boston: Allyn & Bacon.

Fitts, W. H. (1965). *Tennessee self-concept scale manual.* Nashville, Tenn.: Counselor Recordings and Tests, Department of Health.

Flynn, J., & Heffron, P. (1984). *Nursing from concept to practice.* Bowie, Md.: Robert J. Brady.

Gale, R. (1969). *Developmental behavior: A humanistic approach.* London: Collier-MacMillan.

Hames, C. (1978). A theoretical framework for pediatric care: Adaptation-level theory. In P. Brandt (Ed.), *Current practice in pediatric nursing.* St. Louis: C. V. Mosby.

Heffron, P. B., (1984). General systems theory and adaptation. In Flynn, J., & Heffron, P. (Eds.), *Nursing from concept to practice.* Bowie, Md.: Robert J. Brady.

Helson, H. (1964). *Adaptation-level theory.* New York: Harper & Row, Pub.

Kim, H. (1983). *The nature of theoretical thinking in nursing.* Norwalk, Conn.: Appleton-Century-Crofts.

Luckmann, J., & Sorenson, K. (1974). *Medical-surgical nursing: A psychophysiologic approach.* Philadelphia: Saunders.

Phipps, W., Long, B., & Woods, N. (1983). *Medical-surgical nursing concepts and clinical practice.* St. Louis: C. V. Mosby.

Rambo, B. (1984). *Adaptation nursing—Assessment and intervention.* Philadelphia: Saunders.

Roy, C. (1970). Adaptation: A conceptual framework for nursing. *Nursing Outlook, 18*(3), 42.

Roy, C. (1971). Adaptation: A basis for nursing practice. *Nursing Outlook, 19*(4), 254.

Roy, C. (1973). Adaptation: Implications for curriculum change. *Nursing Outlook, 21*(3), 163.

Roy, C. (1976). *Introduction to nursing: An adaptation model.* Englewood Cliffs, N.J.: Prentice-Hall.

Roy, C. (1980). The Roy adaptation model. In J. Rhiel & C. Roy (Eds.), *Conceptual models for nursing practice* (2nd ed.). New York: Appleton-Century-Crofts.

Stevens, B. J. (1984). *Nursing theory—Analysis, application and evaluation* (2nd ed.). Boston: Little, Brown.

The great law of culture is: Let each become all that he was created capable of being.

Thomas Carlyle

2

Culture

Upon completion of the following reading and suggested exercises, the student will be able to:

1. Define the terms *culture, subculture, ethnocentrism,* and *stereotyping.*
2. List and explain the seven characteristics of culture.
3. Describe values and behaviors that are exhibited as a result of cultural experience.
4. Explore and describe cultural variations in beliefs about birth.
5. Discuss the importance of developing a nonjudgmental, sensitive attitude toward people from different cultures.

It is a well-known fact that cultural background affects values, beliefs and, consequently, behavior. Knowledge of a person's sociocultural background is an absolute necessity if a helper is to be optimally effective. It is even more apparent that, with increasingly sophisticated technology in communication, increased availability of travel, and continued social reforms, people of different cultures are working and living closer together. Certainly in America,

We would like to acknowledge the contributions of Jane Fanning, who wrote this chapter in the first edition of *Basic Concepts of Helping.*

with our diversity of people from various subcultures who have retained some aspects of their traditional cultures, there is more need today than ever before to understand, appreciate, and accept individuals of all cultures.

As helpers with a goal of establishing effective helping relationships with clients, you need a receptive, interested, and flexible attitude that will lead you closer to nonjudgmental acceptance of those with diverse sociocultural backgrounds. For example, it is not unusual on a college campus to attend classes with students from all over the world. A student from India could be sitting next to you dressed in very different attire from the traditional "preppy" look seen so frequently on American campuses. Those of us interested in helping must develop warm, friendly, welcoming attitudes toward people who are different from us. Learning to accept people as they are, without passing judgment on their values and behaviors, is a goal of all professional helpers.

The concept of culture and examples of cultural effects on behavior will be discussed in this chapter. As the unit continues, you will learn of the difficulties in acquiring a nonjudgmental attitude and some constructive ways to help you effectively overcome barriers to cultural understanding.

DEFINITION OF CULTURE

Anthropologists are scientists who study culture. Their concepts of culture refer to the values, behaviors, and accepted ways of thinking of a given group of people. They include those behaviors that are learned by means of language and imitation (Barnow, 1971). Edward Tylor (1832–1917), a British anthropologist, is credited with documenting the first definition of culture in his work *Primitive Culture*. He explains it as "that complex whole which includes knowledge, belief, art, law, morals, custom, and any other capabilities and habits acquired by man as a member of society" (Tylor, 1871, p. 1). Through the development of anthropology as a social science, other definitions of culture have evolved. In fact, many books and several hundred definitions of culture have been written by anthropologists (Leininger, 1967).

CHARACTERISTICS OF CULTURE

Many authors have identified the characteristics of culture. For the purpose of this discussion, consider the following seven characteristics:

1. Culture is a group's blueprint for acceptable ways of thinking and behaving.
2. Though culture is universal in human experience, culture is unique for each group of individuals.
3. Culture is transmitted from generation to generation by language and imitation.

4. Culture is stable but continuously adapting.
5. Culture is affected by environment, including such variables as climate, geographical location, food availability, and natural resources.
6. Culture does not affect a person's basic physiological needs (such as need for food or water), but people from different cultural groups may vary genetically.
7. All cultures have four components in common: art forms, language, institutions, and technology.

The following is an in-depth discussion of the previously listed characteristics of culture.

1. *Culture is a group's blueprint for acceptable ways of thinking and behaving.* A blueprint is a plan to guide action, such as the plan for building a house. Culture in this sense is a group's plan for action, or accepted ways of behaving. For example, the cultural group teaches individuals, both overtly and covertly, how to respond to pain. Does the man who has cut his leg in a hunting expedition "keep a stiff upper lip" with little or no response to the injury, or is he encouraged to weep and wail loudly, chant noisily, and refuse to go on with the hunt? The many and varied responses to pain are learned and influenced by the behaviors of individuals within the cultural group. Members of the group are expected to behave to a greater or lesser degree as the group believes.

Zbrowski (1960), in a now classic study, compared the pain responses of Jewish, Italian, and "Old American" patients. He found that the Jewish and Italian patients responded to pain with outward emotion. "Old Americans" tended to be much less emotional in response.

Each culture influences the tangible and intangible things that are valued—attitudes, habits, customs, and laws, to name a few. Culture provides us the blueprint or guide for group acceptability.

2. *Each culture is unique.* All of humanity experiences culture, but no two groups have exactly the same cultural features (Leininger, 1967). For example, all cultures have the need to communicate verbally and nonverbally with one another. But cultures are unique in that each one communicates differently and distinctly from any other. Even when the main language is the same, dialects may arise because languages change as people migrate and these transported languages change in their turn (Malmstrom, 1966). American English and British English are dialects of the same language. The language or dialect is specific or unique to a group of people who share the same culture and is not duplicated by other cultures.

3. *Culture is transmitted from generation to generation.* Usually, the older generation teaches the younger in both informal and formal ways. You may recall family gatherings when your grandfather told of how things were when he was growing up. Learning the ways of one's culture, however, is a lifelong process. Generally, parents, grandparents, older siblings, and others teach and

guide younger members of the group, in a daily, ongoing process, those behaviors that are acceptable and not acceptable. In more formal ways, schools and other groups are established to transmit specific attitudes and knowledge that are considered especially valuable to the culture's existence. Think about how you learned about holiday traditions in your culture. Catholic and Protestant children are taught to anticipate Christmas as a celebration of the birth of Christ and learn to associate Christmas with the excitement of the giving of gifts, decorating the Christmas tree, and singing Christmas carols. Jewish children learn with equal enthusiasm and excitement about Chanukah, a celebration of the ancient Maccabees' victory over the Syrians. It is marked by lighting candles and is celebrated in part by gift giving. Older members of the cultural group share the customs with younger members by reading or telling stories of traditional celebrations. They also encourage children to participate actively in these events.

4. *Culture is stable but continuously adapting.* More often than not a cultural group tends to remain much the same through generations, but this does not mean that cultures never change and become stagnant. All cultures adapt when the need arises. Events occur that influence a culture to change, either slowly and subtly over time or abruptly with little warning. A slower, more subtle change may occur when a cultural group migrates to a new physical location. The influence and intermingling of two cultural groups cause both cultures to change or adapt. For example, the movement of Puerto Ricans to New York City affects the cultures of both Puerto Ricans and New Yorkers. Gradually the two distinct groups adapt to and accommodate each other. Grocery stores and restaurants featuring native Puerto Rican foods begin to spring up, with both cultural groups enjoying the food. At the same time that recent immigrants continue to speak in Spanish, English is being learned as a second language. More abrupt cultural change occurs during war. One culture is rapidly imposed on another, causing the culture to adapt or change rather quickly. During such crisis times, a state of confusion exists and disorder occurs. In crisis, members of a cultural group may not behave as they would during less conflict-ridden times. Traditional values and behaviors that are normally part of the culture may not be evident or practiced. For example, during World War II many Jewish people dramatically changed their religious practices so as not to be noticed and captured by the German Nazis.

5. *Culture is affected by environment.* Many environmental variables exert an effect on culture. For example, the climate and geographical location may determine certain cultural values or behaviors. A natural disaster such as a drought or a hurricane may abruptly cause a temporary or even permanent change in the way a cultural group behaves. Recall that the Plains Indians of America could no longer endure the effects of drought on their food supply and sought to live elsewhere.

Environment particularly affects the way a group meets its physical needs. Consider the foods we eat. Many cultural groups, for example, have a starchy food in their diet that resembles the American pancake. This may be used in combination with other foods rolled up in it or on top of it. Some of these distinct but similar starchy foods include the Mexican tortilla, the French crêpe, the Chinese egg roll, and the Rhode Island jonnycake. The ingredients of this round, flat starchy food are subject to the availability of ingredients in a particular part of the world, and this is directly related to climate.

Perhaps you can think of the ways climate or geographical location affects the dress of a cultural group. Have you ever thought why Western cowboys wear boots and wide-brimmed hats? Or why women from India wear saris? How does geographical location affect the shelter built by the people of a particular culture? Think of the Alpine cabins built in Switzerland or stilt houses built on low-lying, flood-prone areas. Why do Eskimos have igloos and the residents of New Mexico have adobe houses? How are these shelters affected by geographical location? The environment can markedly influence the ways in which a culture lives.

6. *Culture does not affect basic physiological needs, but genetic variation may occur.* Culture does not affect basic physiological needs of people. All people, no matter where in the world they live, have a physiological need for oxygen. Breathing is not affected by the culture of a person. Likewise, when food is needed as a source of energy, hunger is felt; or thirst is felt if fluid is needed. What the person eats or drinks and how and when he or she does are culturally determined, but the sensations of hunger and thirst are the same for everyone.

Certain cultural groups do vary genetically. This is shown in, and caused by, the differences in their inherited characteristics. An example is variance in skin color, or pigmentation. The pigment melanin gives skin its color. It is thought that the darker skin seen in many ethnic groups protects the individual by screening out excess vitamin D from the sun. Conversely, as a result of the gradual migration to colder climates with fewer sunny days, lighter skin evolved to allow maximum vitamin D absorption through the skin.

It is important for professional helpers to realize that many other biological variations occur in cultural groups. Teachers and other helpers working with children in America should be aware that growth and developmental charts used to assess children's progress were primarily developed according to the norms of Anglo-Saxon American children. These norms are not the same for certain other groups such as Blacks, Asians, or American Indians (Overfield, 1977). Another biological variation is seen in cultural groups where adults have been found to lack a certain enzyme necessary for milk digestion. This frequently results in indigestion (Overfield, 1977). If you are a professional helper giving nutritional counseling, how might this knowledge affect your interaction with a client?

There are many other examples of biological variation, including shape and size of the body, fingerprint type, earwax type, and susceptibility to disease. Research continues to investigate and understand biological variation. Knowledge of these important differences is absolutely necessary if professional helpers, especially those involved in health care, are to be optimally effective.

7. *Cultures have four components in common.* All cultures, despite their

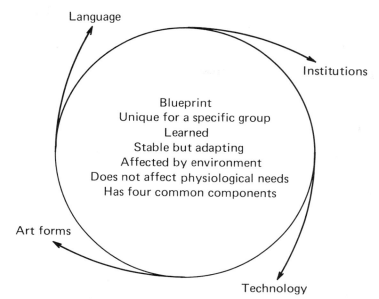

Figure 2-1. The universal experience of culture: its characteristics.

uniqueness, express themselves in four similar ways. They all have art, language, institutions, and technology (Fig. 2–1).

Art is a way to express beauty and emotion and to satisfy one's basic need for self-expression and fulfillment. Art forms include painting or drawing, uses of colors, music, dancing, and so on. Think of the ways you and others in your culture express beauty through art forms. The manner in which you arrange your hair and use makeup is one cultural art form. The rings worn in the noses and ears of some African tribespeople, especially those used to stretch these features, are considered with high regard in these cultures. Music and dancing as art forms are found in all cultures. The popular music of a culture may include symphonic orchestral works or chanting and drum beating. Use of major or minor key may predominate a group's music. The sounds of the sitar, played in India, are quite unlike the sounds of the banjo. Many cultures have forms of musical instruments that are strummed (guitars), blown (horns and pipes), or rhythmically tapped (drums). Art forms are the expressions of a culture's values of beauty and emotion and are passed from generation to generation (Fig. 2–2). The forms seen in a cultural group reflect available natural resources such as the ivory carvings made of elephant tusks from Africa or the baskets woven of reeds from Egypt. Because the perception of beauty is relative, what is considered beauty in one culture may appear to be ugliness in another.

Just as art forms differ between cultures, so they also differ within one culture over time. In pioneer America, pottery served a utilitarian function only. Yet in contemporary America, there are many galleries and local craft

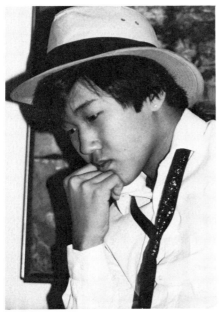

A

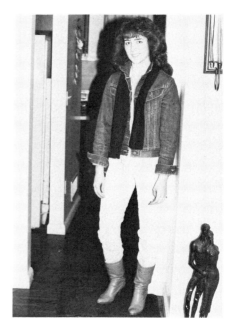

B

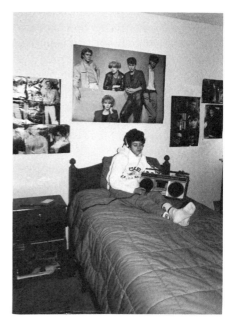

C

Figure 2-2. Art forms of a teen subculture. *(Photo credits to Peggy Haggerty.)*

shows selling and displaying pottery as a form of artistic expression. Dance preferences seem to change dramatically within our American culture. Adolescents of the 1920s learned the Charleston; the 1950s and 1960s brought rock 'n' roll to its peak. And certainly the 1980s will be remembered for break-dancing, begun on the streets of New York City.

All cultures have developed ways to communicate with one another and, indirectly, this helps meet basic needs. We communicate in both verbal and nonverbal ways. For example, language may be of particular relevance to one group, while touching, hand and body movement, and eye contact may have more meaning for another group. Communication methods such as television, satellites, and smoke signals are examples of formal communication channels. Less formal but no less important communication includes chatting, which may occur at the local tavern or at the river bank as women wash the clothing for the family. In fact, sometimes, the quickest way to get news around is through informal channels like the "grapevine." Frequently, however, news traveling via this means loses its reliability!

A professional helper would gain valuable information that could affect the helping relationship if he or she learned the language and communication patterns of the client's group. There are in most languages words that just cannot be translated because they are so unique to that culture. Thus, an occupational therapist working with a predominantly French-speaking clientele would be wise to learn French! Did you know that most children of the world speak two to three languages, while Americans know only one? But even with one main language like English, variations occur within subgroupings of the larger cultural group. American adolescents develop their own meanings for words, like "He's a pothead and all strung out," or "Let's rap." Blacks in Bermuda have developed language patterns that are difficult for visiting Americans to understand because of the fast tempo, even though both Bermudians and Americans speak English. The Navajos are considered polite if they pause and wait before responding to the speaker (Brownless, 1978). In the Hispanic culture, talking with a child without touching the child on the head is thought to mean that the "evil eye" has been cast upon the child. In other cultures, like the British, touch and contact in the form of kissing and hugging is sometimes kept to a minimum, even between parents and children. Many Southeast Asian women avoid eye contact with men when talking to them because it is considered improper to do otherwise.

In summary, all cultures have developed ways to communicate with one another. Learning the subtleties and meanings of nonverbal communication can be very important in establishing effective helping relationships with clients from other cultures. Likewise, learning and using another's language can help to bridge the gap and increase trust between a helper and client from different cultures or subcultures.

All cultures have institutions, or groups of people who live or meet together. The primary purpose of an institution is to meet the social needs of people, including needs for safety, belonging, love, and self-actualization (Maslow, 1954). Institutions provide structure and organization to a culture.

Institutions can be families, religious groups, interest groups, or political groups. Different cultures value certain institutions more than others. Thus, in some cultures, the most valued institution is the family, while in other cultures, the most revered institution is the religious group. Some cultures place such strong emphasis on a particular institution that they become well known for their values. The Amish people are a community people motivated strongly by family tradition. The Soviet society focuses much of its energy on the political state and is strongly identified with that behavior.

Each of us comes from a culture in which certain institutions are of higher priority than others. Can you list three highly valued institutions from your culture?

Technology refers to the equipment or tools that have been developed by a cultural group to help with work and everyday living. Anthropologists have never discovered a cultural group that has not developed its own tools, however primitive. Tools or technology help us to meet our basic needs more effectively or efficiently. In primitive cultures, available natural resources, often in unrefined forms, become the tools for everyday use. Rocks help to grind corn; sticks, logs, and palm fronds are used to build shelter; grasses or animal skins are used for clothing; clays are used to make pottery; native animals are used for transport.

In modern societies, the primitive tools of yesterday are being replaced by more complex technology. Complex machinery mills our flour and makes our bread; synthetic man-made cloth covers our bodies; fiberglass cars transport us; household computers are handling our budgets. Technology is advancing at such a rate that some tools are rapidly rendered obsolete, and it is hard to keep up at times.

It is not uncommon, however, for some members of a culture to cling to the old ways rather than change to the new. Some fields are still plowed by horses; bread is sometimes baked at home. Newer is not necessarily better. The Pennsylvania Amish represent a subculture of Americans who have access to modern conveniences, but prefer to maintain their culture's technology and values as they have been for decades. The elderly frequently reject change—the old ways have served them well for many years.

Helpers need to realize that rejection of new technology is not always negative. There are some traditions that are rich and beautiful and cannot be captured by advanced technology. For example, the arts of calligraphy or hand weaving are irreplaceable. Modern technology has produced more automated approaches and enables us to do wondrous things, but many of the most valuable products, methods, and works of art are those that have been done the "old-fashioned" way.

CONCEPTS RELATED TO CULTURE

To use the concept of culture effectively in professional helping, one must be familiar with several other terms. The first of these is *subculture*.

Subculture

"Subcultures are the small groupings within a culture that have an identity of their own, but are at the same time related to the total culture in certain respects" (Leininger, 1967, p. 31). Research indicates that frequently there are more differences within a given culture than between cultures. Henderson and Primeaux (1981) emphasize that although ethnic characteristics (language, custom, heritage) are important, social class differences determine people's behavior sometimes more than ethnic background. The identifiable differences within a cultural group are the essence of subculture. Members of a subculture may, for example, be of the same age, location, socioeconomic status, and have the same goals, education, occupation, or religion. Protestants, Spanish Americans, adolescents, and New Englanders are subcultures of American society. List the subcultures to which you belong. Keep in mind that, by contrast with *subculture*, the term *culture* refers to the larger grouping. For example, the culture of New Englanders is American (Fig. 2–3). It is vital that helpers know the similarities and the differences of people within a culture, for each is unique within his or her group.

As you learn to become a professional helper, you will find that you must adjust to a new professional subculture. If you are going into the health care field, perhaps as a nurse or a pharmacist, a new subculture you must learn about is that of the health care delivery system. You will learn a whole new language and belief system unique to health care professionals. You will learn new terminology and share in the belief that high-level adaptation and health are valued. If you are going to be a teacher, you will have to learn about the subculture of the educational system of the United States. As you spend time in your educational program, you will gradually assimilate that subculture in which you plan to work. You will become "socialized" into that field.

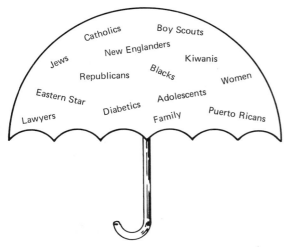

Figure 2-3. All these subcultures come under the umbrella of American culture.

Recognizing differences within a culture also will encourage you to be alert for individual differences. For example, if you are a dental hygienist working with a small boy from India and you have heard it said that "Indian women are timid and withdrawn," keep this in mind as you assess the mother's understanding and compliance regarding her son's care. What you have heard may, in fact, turn out to be true; the mother's behavior may be based on a cultural norm. If so, special support and communication skills may be needed. However, this women also may be different from the norm. Your awareness of cultural behaviors and subcultural and individual uniqueness will enhance your helping capability.

Ethnocentrism

Ethnocentrism, a concept closely related to culture, is the unconscious or conscious tendency for a person to think his or her own culture is superior to that of others. Believing that our culture is superior to others is necessary for survival as a culture. Put simply, we all root for our own team. Recall how you felt watching the most recent Olympics on television. Even though you did not know a single athlete or ever participate in a featured sport, you may have felt a sense of pride and support for your country's team. You cheered for them alone in your own living room because you wanted them to win, to be the best in the world. A phrase like "black is beautiful" is an example of a group's belief in its own worth. In this instance ethnocentrism enhances group members' opinions of themselves and strengthens group cohesiveness.

It is very important for professional helpers to recognize, understand, and accept their own ethnocentric ideas. Although it is idealistic to think that you can view another culture with total objectivity, as a professional helper you must attempt to foster maximum objectivity in yourself to enhance the helping relationship. To force or even share your opinions, biases, beliefs or advice (ethnocentric ideas) upon another will frequently keep a helping relationship from developing. The focus in any helping relationship must be on the client and not on the helper.

The following is an example of a student teacher, Cathy Raye, who allowed her personal biases and ethnocentric ideas to interfere with her helping effectiveness. See if you can pick out her biases in the report she submitted after a visit to Johnny's home. The student teacher is a white Anglo-Saxon Protestant; the client is a white first-generation Spanish-American.

> Johnny B., my pupil, was dressed in a raggedy shirt and pants and watched television throughout the visit. Mrs. B., chewing gum and smoking incessantly, looked unkempt. Her hair was messy, and she wore an old bathrobe and no slippers. Dinner was cooking on the stove and smelled heavily of spices. The house was a mess—old newspapers were on the floor, opened cans and bottles stood on the kitchen shelves, and there were holes in the living room couch and chair. There were no books or magazines evident in the house to encourage reading. In order

to enhance Johnny's reading ability, my advice to Mrs. B. was to: (1) read to Johnny; (2) not allow him to watch television; (3) take Johnny to the library once a week; (4) buy Johnny a magazine subscription to a children's magazine; (5) consider buying an encyclopedia. I left Mrs. B. by saying that with these ideas I felt certain she could help Johnny pull up his grades in reading.

After reading this report, how helpful do you think the student teacher was? Do you think the mother accepted her advice? If you were Mrs. B., would you have followed the student teacher's advice? Why or why not? What could the student teacher have done to more effectively help Johnny and Mrs. B.? Undoubtedly, you can see that the student viewed Johnny and Mrs. B. from her biased ethnocentric frame of reference. She assumes, for example, that Mrs. B. can read. She also assumes that Johnny always watches television. She further thinks this is a poor practice and that a child cannot learn to read if he watches television. She assumes Mrs. B. has a car or other transportation easily accessible or affordable and can easily take Johnny to the library. She further assumes that Mrs. B. and Johnny want to go to the library to improve his reading skills and have the money for the encyclopedia. Obviously, the student was forcing her value system upon her clients without considering where the clients were in their frame of reference.

Certainly becoming a professional helper does not mean you have to give up your own personal ethnocentric behaviors, your strongly held beliefs and values, or your opinions. But you must recognize that you bring your own ethnocentrism with you. You are a product of your culture. You must make a significant attempt to recognize your own ethnocentric behaviors (since most people are unaware of them), thus furthering your understanding of others' ethnocentric behaviors. Strive to be as objective as possible when helping clients.

Stereotyping

Another term related to the concept of culture is *stereotyping*. This is the tendency to say that any one characteristic is typical of all members of a cultural group. Often stereotyped remarks are hastily drawn opinions and prejudgments about a person based on his or her cultural background and do not allow complete understanding of a client as an individual (Fig. 2–4). Stereotyping phrases you may recognize are: "Italian men are sexy," "Southerners are slow and lazy," "Elderly people are forgetful and unreliable," and "Farmers are hardworking." It is amazing how often one characteristic is used to describe all members of a cultural or subcultural group. Can you think of other examples?

One of the dangers in stereotyping is developing group prejudices. Prejudice is destructive to helping relationships. Professional helpers are not expected to like everyone they help, but they must accept them and respect their uniqueness. Care must be taken to avoid creating ethnic stereotypes and generalizations that do not leave room for individual differences. All people

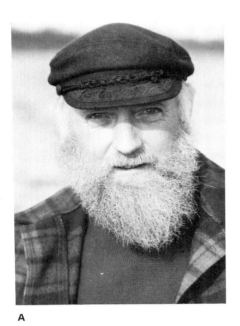

A

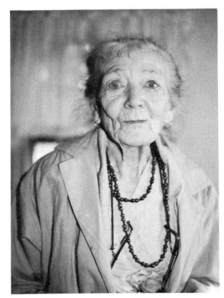

B

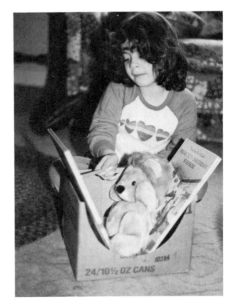

C

Figure 2-4. People make the world go around. Can you identify any common stereotypes about the cultures depicted? **(A)** Where does this man live? Near the sea? **(B)** Elderly people are often labeled "confused." What do you think? **(C)** What do little girls grow up to be? *(Photo credits to Peggy Haggerty.)*

are different, and it is counterproductive to treat all clients alike. What would the consequences be, for example, if every professional helper said, "Unemployed fathers make poor parents"? Stereotyping behavior can inflict great harm on a developing relationship. The client may, because of individual variation, be quite atypical of the entire group. Or your opinion of a group may be very different from the reality. Social scientists have studied many cultural and subcultural groups and have compiled multiple listings of behaviors that are likely to occur in each group. Even though these observations may have been borne out by scientific studies, it is well for the helper not to generalize or stereotype the behavior of the client without additional assessment of the individual's behavior.

Culture Shock

Occasionally, professional helpers work with clients who are experiencing *culture shock*. Kramer (1974) defines this as a "state of anxiety precipitated by the loss of familiar signs and symbols of social intercourse, when one is suddenly immersed in a cultural system markedly different from his own" (p. 4). Culture shock is a temporary condition. Persons experiencing it may be frightened, immobilized, and alone. Because the environment is so foreign to them, they are unable to relate well and communicate effectively. They may retreat into themselves. Certainly, anyone who has traveled to a foreign country has had a taste of what this uncomfortableness feels like. Refugees frequently experience overwhelming loss and depression. But professional helpers are exposed to much less dramatic forms of culture shock . . . and it must be recognized as such. A young child being put on a bus and sent to school for the first time may experience culture shock. A patient admitted to a hospital may find that being immersed in that subculture is frightening and foreign. An aging woman who must sell a house, retain few possessions, and enter a nursing home may experience confusion and depression.

Culture shock is predictable, and there are creative interventions that professional helpers can take to minimize its effects. It must be remembered that those experiencing it are vulnerable and in need of special support—at least temporarily.

CULTURAL VARIATIONS AND SELECTED LIFE EVENTS

All people, regardless of their cultural affiliations, share some life experiences— for example, birth, illness, education, aging, and death. Because these are new to an individual or are stress producing, professional help may be needed. This cross-cultural survey of birth will illustrate a wide range of "normal" or acceptable behaviors. Note that behaviors perceived in one group as normal may be viewed by those in another group as bizarre or totally unacceptable. Awareness of this knowledge is essential for helpers, lest we fall into the same pattern—that is, viewing behaviors of a person from a culture other than ours as bizarre when, in fact, that person is behaving normally according to his or her cultural upbringing.

Birth

In all people the world over the physiological process of conception, pregnancy, and birth occurs in the same way. Yet many of the behaviors surrounding the procreation of the species are culturally determined, and behaviors vary markedly from group to group. Childbearing is viewed as anything from a normal, natural process accomplished solely by the mother to a high risk situation requiring medical or surgical intervention by a team of specially trained doctors.

To traditional Mexicans, pregnancy is desired as soon after marriage as possible. If it does not occur in a year, a . . . special prayer series may be offered. During a first pregnancy (when the pattern for subsequent pregnancies is believed to be determined), there are certain rules and taboos to which this group closely adheres. Cold morning air is considered dangerous both in pregnancy and the postpartum period. Mexican women have a tremendous faith in the goodness of God and God's will being the determining outcome of the birth. Therefore, they tend to have great confidence in their ability to birth. A new mother stays in bed for 3 days, walks around the house after a week, and may venture outside after 2 weeks. In order to avoid cold air, bathing is discouraged and an abdominal binder called a "faja" is worn to prevent an infection. Mexican infants are not breast-fed until after the third day when lactation begins and they traditionally wear a belly band, "fajita," until after the navel heals. Baby girls frequently have their ears pierced (Artschwager, 1978).

Vietnamese women generally marry young and desire large families with many sons. In many families bearing a son—especially a firstborn—gains the wife respect from her in-laws. Vietnamese elders experience considerable esteem, authority, and power, especially if they are men. Men do not attend childbirth. During pregnancy, "unclean" foods such as beef, dog, and snake are avoided. Medical advice, when needed, is usually sought from herbalists, who play a significant role in Vietnamese folk medicine.

The Vietnamese believe that much body heat is lost during labor and delivery and it must be replaced. Traditionally, this was accomplished by burning a brazier of smoldering wood under the new mother's bed. Today hot herb teas and soups are drunk; cold beverages are avoided. Bathing and shampooing are kept to a minimum, lest they wash away nutrients, heat, and energy. A 1-month rest period after delivery is desirable.

Vietnamese village women generally breastfeed their infants for several years and rarely have them sleep alone. Circumcisions are not acceptable. "Determining the age of a Vietnamese infant can be very confusing since the infant is usually considered to be a year old at birth and becomes another year older at the next Tet, or New Year" (Stringfellow, 1978, p. 180). Neonates are dressed in old clothes and rarely praised, to keep the spirits from finding them desirable and either stealing them or making them ill.

Women of the world differ greatly in the amount of mechanical and human assistance they have during birth. Depending on the culture, the mother may be accompanied by another woman, her mother, the father of the baby, or perhaps a whole group of people. In some cultures the attendants touch the mother—massaging her abdomen and rubbing her back—encouraging her, making birth a social event. This touching varies from light touch to very rough and violent abdominal shaking. Music may be used to relax the mother, and various salves, including butter and root juices, are used as lubricants to the massage. In the Yucatan, rupturing uterine membranes is considered dangerous and unnatural, while in the United States many obstetricians find this a useful and routinely advisable practice. Attendants in both the Yucatan and the United States are using methods appropriate for their particular cultural system and are acting in the best interests of mother and child as the practice is culturally defined.

Canadian and Soviet women usually receive their maternity care from a team of highly specialized doctors and nurses. This is certainly contrary to the home birthing with nurse midwives that is familiar to British and Scandinavian women. In the People's Republic of China high-technology assessment of fetal well-being is emphasized as couples strive to have a perfect infant. Due to the large population, birth control is promoted: one-child families are rewarded, while larger ones are penalized. If fetal testing reveals a less than perfect infant, an abortion is commonly obtained.

Cultural groups view eating and drinking during labor differently. For example, the Yumans of North America developed strong prohibitions against drinking water during labor. They believe that the mother would die if she drank during labor. In Great Britain, eating and drinking during labor are not prohibited but are, in fact, encouraged. Light meals are given to keep up the mother's strength. In all cultures a reason is given to justify practice, and the reason may be scientifically based and provable, or mystical or spiritual. In any case, the reason given seems to be believed, accepted, and practiced by the members of the group.

Recall that one of the characteristics of culture is that it is dynamic and adaptive. The American way of childbearing is evolving even now. Most women in the 1940s were anesthetized during late labor and delivery. They were, therefore, not aware of their babies' births until much later, frequently after fathers and family members had been notified! During the 1960s a prepared childbirth movement began that greatly affected the childbearing options available to women of the 1980s. Parents began to assert themselves and demand fuller participation. Fathers insisted upon their rights to be present when their children were born. Childbirth education classes sprang up all over America, attended by thousands of expectant, interested parents. Infants today are healthier. Mothers require less medication. Both suffer fewer complications. Independent birthing centers, nurse-midwife attendants, and sibling participation have gained in popularity. Interestingly, an increasing number of women have been giving birth in an upright position. This is quite different from the back-lying position encouraged by the medical technology of the past decades. Ironically, it is similar to the age-old squat that Third World women have always used to make the best use of gravity!

Most American women in the past 50 years have chosen to bottle-feed, even though the American Academy of Pediatrics has stated that breast-feeding is the desirous method. Unfortunately, the bottle-feeding practice has negatively influenced other cultures that attempt to pattern themselves after America and are vulnerable to its advertising. Hundreds of African and other Third World babies born in the past 10 years have had gastrointestinal illnesses as a result of consumption of improperly sterilized formulas diluted with contaminated water supplies. Thus, a health problem has arisen in one culture as a result of its attempt to assimilate the life-styles of another culture.

While Americans shun breast-feeding, others advocate it. Filipino women are expected to breast-feed and do so. Its value is highly regarded.

TOWARD NONJUDGMENTAL HELPING

Professional helpers need to expand their appreciation of the cultural dimensions of their clients. To ignore this is to alienate the person. Clark (1978) points out that:

> Individuals under stress . . . tend to place considerable reliance on cultural patterns as a method of coping. Indeed, magical and religious practices can be psychotherapeutic in that they can bring about the social support of the community of persons of like culture. (p. vii)

Thus, utilizing one's knowledge of a client's cultural background can facilitate the helping relationship.

A professional helper faces the difficult task of developing a nonjudgmental, sensitive, accepting attitude toward others' culturally determined behaviors (Fig. 2–5). Even once understanding of another's culturally induced values and beliefs has occurred, it may be difficult or even impossible for many reasons to help the person effectively. However, understanding culture does remove one possible barrier to establishing an effective helping relationship.

The person you are helping should not ever feel that what is said will be held against him or her. In a helping relationship, a client who has a strong religious belief or takes a radical political stand should never feel as though the sharing of personal ideas will be unjustly judged by the helper. The helper must accept the fact that people have different values and beliefs and allow the client full freedom in the helping relationship to express these beliefs. The helper maintains a neutral stand, while allowing and encouraging the client

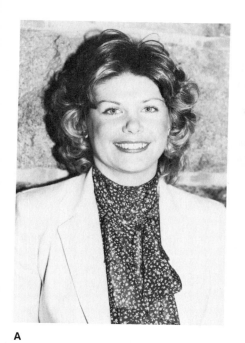

A

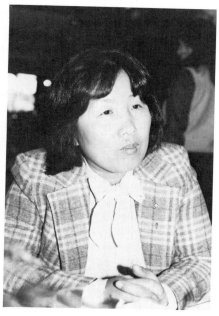

B

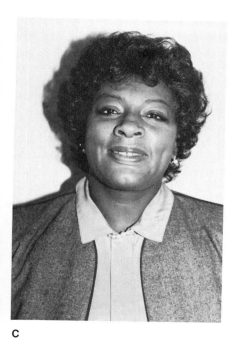

C

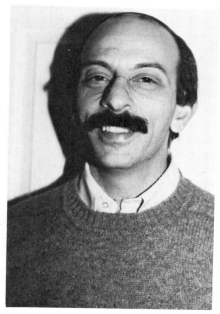

D

Figure 2-5. Faces of culture. Sensitivity and open-mindedness are essential to the understanding of a cultural group different from your own. *(Photo credits to Peggy Haggerty.)*

to discuss values and behave according to culturally instilled beliefs. It is the helper who must remain flexible, nonjudgmental, and open. Consider this situation:

> You are a public health nurse visiting a young Spanish-speaking mother in a large city barrio. You notice that the grandmother of the baby is giving most of the care and, although the temperature is 90° F in the home, the baby's head and ears are covered with a cap. Your first instinct might be to tell the mother the baby does not need the cap; it is too warm. This is your belief, and you can give scientific reasons why this cap is unnecessary.

The astute helper realizes there might be another belief held by the mother and grandmother—which is, in fact, true. They believe the cap keeps bad air away from the baby. To try to change this behavior would be unnecessary and contribute to loss of security for the mother. Do you see that a helper who forces personal values on a client could harm or hinder a relationship rather than help it?

There will be times when the helper realizes that a strongly held belief could be a dangerous or an unsafe practice. The mother cited above also uses a raisin on the open umbilical cord of her baby to keep out bad air. If you think this might be causing an umbilical infection, you must attempt to gain the mother's trust before attempting to change behavior. It takes great skill to change firmly held beliefs!

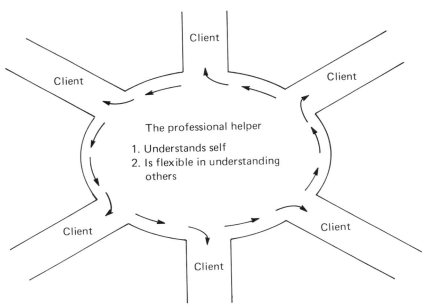

Figure 2-6. The helper interacts with clients from varied sociocultural groups.

As Figure 2–6 shows, it is the professional helper who is the pivotal or flexible one in the relationship. The helper must first understand his or her own beliefs, cultural biases, and values. Once this is accomplished, the helper can, with more freedom and flexibility, adapt to and understand the ways of others. The helper will be in a better position to recognize the sources of discrepancy. The goal is to get as close to understanding another's culture as possible. If this means experiencing the culture firsthand, which might be appropriate in some cases, then consider learning the native language or visiting in homes and communities. Always be open to increasing your understanding of the more subtle aspects of another's culture.

Helping others who come from different cultural backgrounds does not have to be a frustrating experience and one to be avoided. Rather, the well-prepared helper equipped with knowledge of others' cultural background and having skills to work with others effectively can succeed in establishing maximally helpful and satisfying relationships. Simultaneously, the helper can gain and grow a great deal too!

CONCLUSION

In this chapter you have considered ways in which understanding the concept of culture can enhance your work as a nonjudgmental professional helper. You have attempted to understand your own cultural background as well as the cultural heritage of others. You have considered the consequences on the helping relationship if the helper does not attempt to understand the cultural differences of others.

Today, as never before, distances between far points in the world seem closer. Vastly different cultural groups are no longer separated by oceans or mountains. Supersonic jetliners traverse the span between Paris and New York in less than 4 hours. Only 35 years ago the same flight took 16 hours. And it took the Pilgrims almost 3 months to travel the same distance in 1620. Advanced technology has brought cultures together. People, especially professional helpers, must become actively involved in bridging cultural gaps and increasing understanding among fellow human beings.

IMPORTANT REMINDERS

1. The concept of culture includes those learned values, beliefs, and behaviors that are a result of association with a given group of people.
2. Cultures have the ability to adapt over time, yet each is unique from all others. Culture is expressed through art, technology, institutions, and language.
3. Professional helpers need to understand and accept the variations that people have as individuals. Basic to this is a sense of self-awareness and an ability to be objective and nonjudgmental.

REFERENCES

Artschwager, K. M. (1978). The Mexican American. In A. Clark (Ed.), *Culture, child-bearing, and health professionals*. Philadelphia: Davis, pp. 88–109.

Barnow, V. (1971). *An introduction to anthropology*. Homewood, Ill.: Dorsey Press.

Brownless, A. T. (1978). *Community, culture, and care*. St. Louis: C. V. Mosby.

Clark, A. (Ed.). (1978). *Culture, childbearing, and health professionals*. Philadelphia: Davis.

Henderson, G., & Primeaux, M. (1981). *Transcultural health care*. Menlo Park, Calif.: Addison-Wesley.

Kramer, M. (1974). *Reality shock*. St. Louis: C. V. Mosby.

Leininger, M. (1967, April). The culture concept and its relevance to nursing. *Journal of Nursing Education, 6,* 27–37.

Malmstrom, J. (1966, Winter). Dialects. *The Florida Reporter.*

Maslow, A. (1954). *Motivation and personality*. New York: Harper & Row.

Overfield, T. (1977, March). Concepts from physical anthropology. *Nursing Clinics of North America 12* (1). Philadelphia: Saunders, pp. 19–26.

Stringfellow, L. (1978). The Vietnamese. In A. Clark (Ed.), *Culture, childbearing, and health professionals*. Philadelphia: Davis, pp. 174–182.

Tylor, E. (1871) *Primitive culture: Researches into the development of mythology, philosophy, religion, language, art, custom*. New York: Holt, Vol. I, p. 1.

Zbrowski, M. (1960). Cultural components in response to pain. In D. Apple (Ed.), *Sociological studies of health and sickness*. New York: McGraw-Hill.

We have learned that we cannot live alone. . . . We have to be citizens of the world, members of the human community.

Franklin Delano Roosevelt

3

Group

Upon completion of this reading and suggested exercises, the student will be able to:
1. Define a group.
2. Identify four types of groups.
3. Describe the effects that size, composition, format, and environment have on group functioning.
4. Name and briefly explain the task and maintenance functions necessary for an effective group.
5. Identify the four phases of group development and compare these to the psychosocial development of the person.
6. Describe the components of responsible membership in a group.
7. Recognize behaviors that are disruptive to group effectiveness.
8. Describe the characteristics of an effective group leader.
9. Explain the importance of gaining strong skills in group theory and dynamics as a beginning professional helper.

Our society has become dominated by group interactions. It is rare for any individual to work alone. Most people depend upon and work with others in some form of group structure. As helpers, you will find that expanded knowledge of group process will help you in your work with clients and colleagues. A cohesive group structure can serve as a very productive model assisting you in your work as a professional helper.

There is seemingly no end to the number of groups in our society. In the past decade groups have proliferated! Think for a moment of the numbers of people getting married, having families, or entering housing for the elderly. It is quite likely that these people have joined temporary groups to prepare them for marriage and/or for the birthing of a child, or more permanent groups such as a housing association to help them with daily living problems. Many people have joined the collectives and cooperatives that have recently emerged: women's health groups, food cooperatives, farm collectives (kibbutzim), condominiums, and similar associations.

Everyone has had experiences with and belonged to both temporary and permanent groups. Consider for a moment only those groups to which you belong. First, you originate in a family. You are probably a student and also may be employed. Therefore, you belong to a business or occupational group and may associate with a subgroup. Perhaps you participate in a religious or recreational group. Are you a member of a social club or fraternity? How about organizations? Are you on any committees within these organizations? Can you identify the permanent groups to which you belong? The temporary groups? What are your commitments to both types of groups? Are they different?

DEFINITION AND PURPOSE OF A GROUP

A group can be defined as two or more individuals united frequently in repeated interaction for a common purpose. This common purpose generally is to share an interest or task, resolve a problem, or fulfill a mutual need. Groups are a fundamental unit of human existence. Although the family is considered one's primary group because of its significance and influence, each person belongs to several groups. Though these groups differ in their functioning and objectives, all of them have a purpose. For optimal group effectiveness, members must feel a sense of unity toward that purpose, and all must work to attain it.

For example, if you decide to join the swim team, it is a requirement that each member be committed to certain responsibilities—attending practices on time and swimming a required number of laps per day. Members who do not follow the team rules can ruin the experience for every member. Entire governments have collapsed when large groups of the population have changed their focus of behavior. When a group is mature and effective, its membership shares that common purpose with a sense of togetherness. They feel that the purpose is rational and attainable by the group. They feel that, at least in one respect, they have commonality with one another.

TYPES OF GROUPS

As we have seen, groups may be distinguished as either temporary or permanent, depending upon how long they are in existence to achieve a purpose. The makeup of the membership also will influence the life expectancy of a given group. With a changing membership, a given group may go on indefinitely, since new members are continually joining.

Groups also can be differentiated according to the general purpose they serve. Combs, Avila, and Purkey (1971), for example, have identified four classifications of groups most commonly used by professional helpers:

- Conversational—typified by the "bull session" which has a high degree of participation. Descriptive dialogue, friendly rapport, and strong interpersonal compatibility predominate. Its prototype may be seen in the family or social group.
- Instructional—designed so that a leader can verbally and/or visually demonstrate something to the group. Members share a need to learn something, such as assertiveness or how to stop smoking or how to become a professional helper.
- Decision—oriented toward decision making and problem solving using basic communication skills of sharing, listening, and questioning. City governments, boards of directors, collectives, and businesses are all dependent upon this type of group functioning.
- Discovery utilizes the group process to assist members in self-awareness and disclosure, as they simultaneously explore and discover their relationship to their environment (p. 279). Thus, members learn intrapersonal as well as interpersonal skills. In this type of group a supportive atmosphere and a highly skilled, empathetic, perceptive leader are essential. Some familiar forms of this group include sensitivity training, group therapy, and learning groups.

GROUP CHARACTERISTICS

Thus, a group evolves when any number of people unite for a common cause. Many of these groups are related to the work of professional helpers. Many groups are actually initiated by professional helpers. When this occurs, it is frequently the professional who accepts ultimate accountability and responsibility for seeing that the cause or purpose is achieved. To be most effective, the helper must understand group structure, function, and process. These are

STRUCTURE	Size Composition Format Physical environment	**Process Phases** Formative Developmental Working Termination	Task Maintenance	FUNCTIONS

Figure 3-1. Group characteristics.

the three basic components of characteristics of a group. Figure 3–1 elaborates on these, as does the following discussion.

Group Structure

Group structure refers to the framework for the group. It is the arrangement of the elements, the setting of the stage. This is not to imply that structure is permanent. It may, and does, change as group needs change. But if a group is to be effective, appropriate planning and thought must determine its structure. Structure includes group size and composition, physical environment, and group format. For example, if you belong to a hockey team, you know there will be 11 other players, a preplanned schedule of games to play, a coach, and three 15-minute periods in which to win.

Size and Composition.   Probably the single most important consideration in determining the optimal size of a group is knowledge of its purpose or objective. The techniques that will be used to accomplish that objective will be determined by, and dependent upon, the group size. Groups that have as an objective decision making or psychotherapy, for example, should be small. Recreational groups and community action groups may be enhanced by having larger memberships.

Size can have a pronounced effect upon the ability of a group to function (Fig. 3–2). While the literature is inconsistent in its recommendations regarding the optimal size of a group, some interesting findings have been reported. Yalom and Terrazas (1968) suggest that a group needs at least four or five active members to be productive. It stands to reason that as this number decreases to one or two, the pressure upon these more involved members increases. Other authors such as Coffey (1966) have warned about the dangers of a group becoming an assemblage. It appears that this is likely to occur most frequently when the number of people meeting together approaches 16 to 20. Sampson and Marthas (1977) report that observation and evaluation of members becomes increasingly difficult as the membership surpasses 7. Marram (1978) summarizes that the:

> . . . usual size of a small group for therapeutic purposes should be 6–10 individuals plus the leader . . . it is felt that any more (or less) in the group will inhibit the kind of feedback exchange desired to promote client self-awareness. (p. 150)

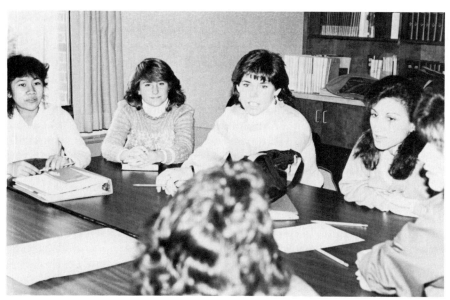

A

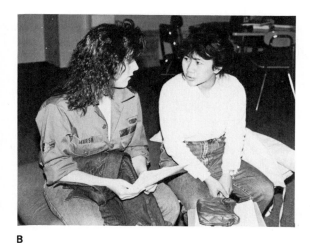

B

Figure 3-2A and B. Groups consist of two or more people. Remember it is responsible membership that makes a group work. *(Photo credits to Peggy Haggerty.)*

Vinter (1967) summarizes that:

> Large groups (e.g., nine or over) tend toward anonymity of membership, higher demands for leadership abilities . . . small groups, in contrast, tend toward high rates of member participation, greater individual involvement, greater consensus, and increased restraint upon members. Relations among persons in smaller groups tend to be more intensive, other things being equal. (p. 35)

In addition, it has been suggested that as the size of a group increases, there is an increasing tendency for lower member satisfaction (Sampson & Marthas, 1977). "Most insight, or talk oriented groups, seem to function best with 6–10 members. This is also a good size for instructional groups in which the members need time and assistance to practice new skills," like Lamaze groups or skiing classes (Loomis, 1979, p. 61).

The composition of a group can greatly enhance or inhibit its effectiveness regardless of size. Composition refers to the group members' characteristics. In open groups—those in which membership is constantly changing—composition cannot be as readily controlled as in closed groups with consistent membership. Whenever possible, however, care should be taken to compose groups whose members are compatible so that one or more does not have reason to be isolated or feel "different." It may, for example, be uncomfortable to be the only female in an otherwise all-male group, the only black, the only shy and quiet person, the only beginner, the only over-40-year-old. This factor is particularly important in small groups and discovery groups, which depend most heavily upon supportive interaction of members (Fig. 3–3).

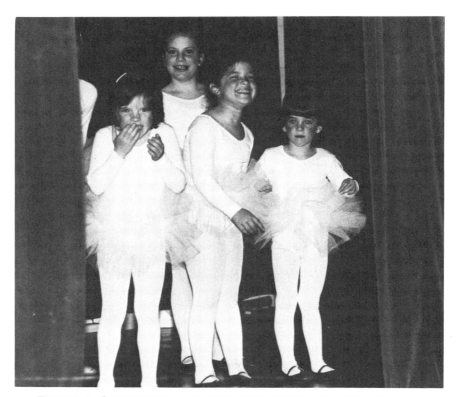

Figure 3-3. Could there be any doubt about the purpose, composition, or potential for growth in this group? *(Photo credit to Mary Logan.)*

Physical Environment.   Careful consideration should be given to selecting the time and place for group meetings. Both should facilitate the membership's involvement.

Timing includes both length of meeting and frequency of contact. A swimming instructor, for instance, may consider offering eight 1-hour classes in a 4-week session twice a week, or in an 8-week series once a week. The instructor may consider such factors as retention of information, time needed for practice, calendar constraints, physical duration versus exhaustion, and concentration ability. Certainly, timing should be convenient for all group members.

Members need to be responsible about time commitments, and leaders need to make sure meetings do not go beyond their expected time. A designated time frame should be given in advance, and members should not be expected to stay beyond the allotted time. Certainly, there are exceptions to this rule, especially in instances of major discussions. These exceptions, however, should be considered just that—members become frustrated when time commitments are not adhered to.

The physical arrangements for a group must be carefully planned around the group's purpose. Room size, lighting, comfort level, location, and esthetics are all crucial factors. Appropriate equipment should be readily available.

Seating arrangements should be thought out—round tables are conducive to discussions, and rows of seats, facing forward are conducive to didactic instruction. If audiovisual material is used, the person responsible for it should be sure the equipment is in working order and ready to use. Valuable meeting time has often been wasted in looking for a new light bulb for the film projector! A room that is too hot, too cold, or noisy can deter group productivity. Certainly plush arrangements are not necessary, but comfortable arrangements are always an asset to group functioning.

Format.   The format of a group refers to the manner and style in which a group conducts itself. It includes the way in which it is internally organized and its members' communication patterns with one another. It is undoubtedly one of the most crucial elements related to a group's success. Perhaps one of the most frustrating experiences is to be in a group that cannot seem to accomplish its task! Frequently all that is needed is a restructuring of members' roles and communication patterns.

Some groups are highly organized systems of authority, and power is delineated with complex job descriptions and role expectations. Others operate quite effectively with similar components that are less rigid. Many decision-making groups progress through an agenda following *Roberts' Rules of Order*. A president or leader presides, and a designated secretary records the minutes for later reference. Still other groups, such as community action groups, offer minimal structure and are totally dependent upon motivated volunteers, frequently operating without a designated leader. The organizational structure that is selected for a group needs to be compatible with its purpose and size. This can either be prearranged by the group's organizer or self-selected at its first meeting.

A group's communication pattern describes "who talks to whom about what" (Loomis, 1979, p. 77). Formally organized groups adhere to strict rules regarding discussion. They describe when a member may talk and to whom comments may be directed. All members are expected to know the rules and follow them or they will be reprimanded and called "out of order." Such groups either discourage free dialogue or carefully monitor it. This is exemplified by the traditional classroom with the teacher as the pivotal figure. Many nations operate their governments in this style. Other groups are most effective if members openly and spontaneously share with one another. In fact, some groups cannot operate at all without openness.

Figure 3–4 demonstrates four basic patterns of group communication. They are the chain, the wheel, the circle, and the sociometric star. Germane to all of them is the concept of centrality. Centrality is "the position of dominance in a communication network from which and through which most communication flows" (McCann-Flynn & Hefron, 1984, p. 577). Note in the figure that the central person in the chain is B, in the wheel E, in the circle no one, and in the star D. Think for a moment about some groups to which you belong (i.e., your family, roommates, a college seminar group or work group). Map out the communication network of each. Do you think each of these groups is maximally achieving its objectives? Would a change in the communication pattern help? You may have noticed that a given group may communicate by using more than one of the basic patterns (note in Figure 3–4 that in the star configuration a chain naturally occurs among A, D, and F). As you might

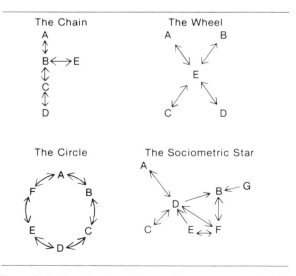

Figure 3-4. Four basic patterns of group communication.

imagine, the communication pattern of a group is the key to its achievement of purpose, and it behooves a leader to be aware of subgroupings within a group!

It is important to realize that communication patterns are not always fixed. Frequently, when certain groups first meet, the circle is helpful for discussion, but when the group finally decides upon a course of action, the wheel is most useful. Consider the following example:

> Five men, Mike, Jim, James, Joshua, and Edward, are renting a small house for their final year in college. Before they agreed to do this, they established certain ground rules about household responsibilities, food preparation, and socializing. Edward has been deviating from the group's expectations. He has not been doing his share of the work.
>
> Mike, John, James, and Joshua meet to talk about the problem and how to approach Edward. The discussion is meaningful, and the group decides that James would be the most tactful in talking to Edward. Hence, the pattern of communication begins to change, and the suggestions of how to handle this problem are directed towards James.

In research comparing the circle, chain, and wheel there are some interesting findings. The results of research by Leavitt (1958) and Smith (1951) indicate that the wheel is the most efficient arrangement for simple problem solving; the chain is next, and the circle is the least efficient. However, as the complexity of the task increases, especially as it requires decision making and evaluation of alternatives, then the circle proves to be the most efficient and the wheel the least efficient. This is particularly true if the central person is not very capable or if the peripheral members with good ideas never get a chance to have them evaluated by others in the group. Also, it appears that with simple tasks, group morale and a sense of satisfaction are highest in the circle, where all are involved, and least high in the wheel, where one member's centrality dominates and leaves the others out of the picture.

The sociometric star, a model originally proposed as a "personality attraction model" (Moreno, 1951, p. 53), is included here since "communication tends to follow the attraction structure; persons linked by liking relationships tend to communicate more with one another" (Sampson & Marthas, 1977, p. 58). Clearly, as a communication pattern, the star shares some of the problems of the wheel.

Group Process

The second major characteristic of a group is its process. This refers to the growth of a group and implies change and adaptation. Group process involves progressive stages of development. While authors differ regarding the particulars, there is general agreement as to the trend of group development. The following is a composite of those views (Bernstein, 1973; Lacoursiere, 1980; Semrad & Arsenian, 1975; Vinter, 1967):

The period of origin, when a group is initiating its activity and orienting its members, is called the *formative stage*. Members frequently have a sense that some good will come out of the group experience, so they are eager and optimistic. On occasion there are members who join groups involuntarily and do not have these positive feelings. Beginning groups generally are dependent upon and seek direction from a designated leader. Superficial relationships are formed, commitment and trust begin, and the group purpose and structure surface. It is normal for members to feel some anxiety and hesitation in this unknown situation, so risk-taking is minimal and guarded interaction is to be expected.

In the *developmental stage*, as the group establishes itself and clarifies its purpose and direction, a normal period of struggle ensues. Members realize that their individual expectations have to be compromised or adjusted to blend with those of other members and of the group as a whole. Frustration, anger, and dissatisfaction result. Individuals or subgroups of individuals may compete with, resist, or dominate one another. Aggression is sometimes directed toward the group leader, and authority or power may be tested. The roles of the leader and members emerge as progress begins toward conflict resolution and accomplishment of the group's purpose. Ultimately, cooperation and cohesion begin, with members having gained an awareness and understanding of one another. This enhances trust development and enables the group to progress to the next stage.

In the *working* or *mature stage* of development there is stabilization of the group's purpose, process, and dynamics. Anxieties and conflicts are replaced with cooperative behavior. Differences of opinion and feeling are viewed as healthy and challenging rather than threatening. Eagerness is rekindled, and one begins to see progress as group needs override individual needs. It is not unusual to note a change in leadership style during this stage. A productive, maturely functioning group may thrive better with distributive leadership that encourages autonomy.

The final stage, *termination*, occurs when group objectives are fulfilled or time limits are met. Groups also may be abruptly interrupted or may disintegrate from a lack of adaptation. Generally, however, there are positive feelings of accomplishment, mixed with regrets at what was not accomplished and sadness in knowing it will all end soon. (You may recall having these feelings most vividly at your high school graduation.)

Group Functions

The third and final characteristic of a group is its function. Much of the research that has been done on groups has focused on the skills and functions that are needed for a group to accomplish its purpose effectively. These are usually categorized as task functions and maintenance functions, categories based upon the original work of Benne and Sheats (1948). The following discussion is partly adapted from that of Bradford (1976) in *Making Meetings Work*.

Task Functions. These functions must be accomplished if the group is to meet its purpose or objective. They emphasize the group as a whole for the purpose of problem solving and include the following:

- Initiate—suggesting how the group might begin; posing an agenda, new questions, suggesting new direction, and defining group problems. Redirecting and reenergizing the discussion as needed throughout the duration of the group's existence.
- Seek information and opinion—requesting facts, ideas, beliefs, and suggestions to assure that group action and decision is firmly based. To get an accurate representation, opinions must be gathered from all of the members.
- Give information and opinion—offering facts, ideas, beliefs, and suggestions which are relevant to the group's concerns. One's ability to do this is dependent "upon sufficient trust, caring and respect for each member, and active listening" (Bradford, 1976, p. 39).
- Clarify/elaborate—restating ideas to validate understanding; interpreting or explaining in different ways with examples to help others clarify their thinking; expanding upon and/or coordinating ideas to enhance their meaning and relevancy. This requires keen listening skills so one can detect when an idea has been half-stated and needs to be questioned or expanded if it is not to be lost. Elaborating and clarifying encourages more timid group members to share when they know someone will help build upon their thoughts.
- Coordinate/summarize—restating ideas or suggestions for review; combining related ideas and stating them in a single integrated form; reviewing where the group has been, where it is now, and where it seems to be going.
- Consensus testing—checking with the group to see if it is nearing agreement or ready for a decision; stating conclusions for the group's acceptance or rejection.

Task functions facilitate a group's progress and are the responsibility of all of its members. Employed appropriately, they will enhance group communication.

Critical in the performance of task functions is the all-important skill of timing. These useful behaviors lose their value if they are used at the wrong time or with the wrong intention.

Maintenance Functions. Functions that facilitate the group process and focus on the group members more directly than on the group purpose are the maintenance functions. They "involve feelings, moods, attitudes, needs, and the growth of individual members and the group as a whole" (Bradford, 1976, p. 42). They include:

- Gatekeeping—facilitating the communication process by encouraging and inviting participation from those members who share less readily and monitoring those that may be dominating the discussion. When more verbal persons dominate, group cohesion and growth stagnate or diminish. "Sensitive gatekeeping is vital to good group morale; without it some members remain isolated and rejected, and potential contributions are lost" (Bradford, 1976, p. 43).
- Encouraging—accepting, supporting, and praising group members and their contributions. Requires sensitivity, perception, empathy, responsiveness, and friendliness. Includes appropriate use of feedback and an openness to differences.
- Harmonizing—attempting to mediate differences or resolve conflicts among group members; reducing tensions, frustration, anger, fighting, etc. May include the use of humor.
- Standard-setting—discussing the group's progress, fairness, maturity, atmosphere, etc. Includes reminding the group of its commitment and asking the members how they feel about the group.

It is the general consensus of opinion among those knowledgeable and skilled in group dynamics that groups are most productive when task and maintenance functions are distributed among the members. That is, all group members should possess skills and assume responsibility. This increases the chance that everyone's assets will be most effectively utilized. It also tends to strengthen the commitment to the group and the member's satisfaction with the group. In the absence of members who are able or willing to assume functions, the group leader must be more visible. It is the leader's responsibility to encourage and facilitate maximum member participation in task and maintenance behaviors. If this fails, the leader must be prepared actually to do these functions alone.

RESPONSIBLE MEMBERSHIP

Basic to the dynamics of any group are the behaviors of its members. Too frequently emphasis is placed on leadership, usually by a single individual. When this happens, it is much too easy to overlook the significance of responsible membership.

> Certain behaviors are expected from a person . . . in a group. . . . Position means the place occupied within the group. Status means the rank or importance of the place occupied. The sum total of these behaviors is called the role. The individual occupying the role must be content with the role

and its social norms and these behaviors must be compatible with the individual's personal needs (Gerrard, Boniface, & Love, 1980, p. 240)

During the development of a group, each individual settles into a role that is appropriate for his or her own needs and experience. This role may change as the group needs change. Each person achieves a balance between personal needs and group needs. Most effective groups have members who are flexible in role change.

Consider Marilyn Ruize, the president of the Parent–Teacher Organization. For 2 years she has been the key person in charge of overseeing most of the extra curricula and fund-raising activities at the school. Although her term of office is up, Marilyn has decided to remain involved, but would prefer a less time-consuming role. Marilyn becomes part of the executive board and in this role advises the new president. For Marilyn, the adjustment from a leadership to a membership role is a welcome change, and she feels that she continues to make an important contribution.

Being a responsible member involves specific behaviors and attitudes. It is, of course, of primary importance that a person feel connected to a group, that there be a reason to be involved, and that he or she feel capable of being an effective member. Without a sense of belonging, one can rarely develop commitment to a group or gain satisfaction from participating in the group.

Once one feels a sense of belonging and purpose, motivation to contribute and share follows. As in learning, internally inspired motivation is a stronger catalyst than externally lured motivation. Ideally, all members of a group want to be involved! Realistically, this does not usually happen, as we all know. Surely you can recall times when you have gone to a meeting, attended an event, or taken a required course in which you did not want to be involved. You probably got out of the experience exactly what you put into it! Thus, responsible membership involves desire and commitment to become actively involved.

Active involvement includes going to meetings on time and being prepared. Any out-of-group assignments should be completed and ready to be shared with others. During the group activities, members should actively participate. If this includes discussion, it is important to listen attentively as well as verbally contribute. Ideas, suggestions, feelings, and questions should be readily shared. It is important to admit confusion promptly and seek clarification so that one's level of involvement does not diminish as the group's progress continues beyond one's ability to participate. A mature group member is knowledgeable regarding the task and maintenance functions needed by the group. The member assists with these whenever able, being careful not to place personal needs and interests before those of the group.

As one recognizes personal strengths and abilities within a given group and responds to the needs of other members, role identity strengthens. Clear expectations help members to avoid disharmony, role confusion, and ambiguity. It also is important not to make any one member accountable for too much. Role overload can be draining and can result in poor-quality performance.

In any kind of group, support and encouragement of other members is important. It builds trust and enhances feelings of self-worth. Friendships grow, and communication and participation are fostered. Thus, all group members should be warm and open with others in the group.

Membership involves accountability. Members are responsible for their own actions and assume active roles in assisting the group to accomplish given tasks. Members must be ready to assume leadership roles, as this often happens informally. Members must, also, be honest about their concerns and share them during group meetings. Frequently, members inappropriately blame poor leadership for a poorly functioning group.

> Consider Hazel Downs, a member of the campaign committee for the local Republicans. A position has become available on the local school board, and Hazel is aware of the fact that a good campaign could easily get a Republican candidate elected. However, John Thomas, the campaign committee chairperson, has not contacted her—so Hazel does nothing about the situation except to complain about John Thomas's poor leadership.

It is the contention of the authors of this book that members have responsibilities, too! Hazel Downs is not responding in a productive, helpful way. What do you think Hazel should do?

Within the role of membership is the notion of individual leadership. Members are not robots who are programmed as to how they should act. Members are creative thinkers who work cooperatively in an effort to accomplish a common goal. Can you think of other instances in which group members should assume more of a leadership role?

DISRUPTIVE PERSONALITIES

One of the most frustrating—and challenging—things a group must contend with is dysfunctional or disruptive behavior in one or more of its members. If this problem is inadequately handled, a few individuals can ruin a group experience and inhibit growth. In most cases, preventive action and thought can avoid unpleasant situations.

> The tighter the leader controls task functions and a few group functions, the greater the amount of dysfunctional behavior in the group. Conversely, when the leader shares responsibility and helps members learn how to control and develop their own group, there is less dysfunctional member behavior. (Bradford, 1976, p. 47)

A sensitive leader will be able to recognize and deal with potentially disruptive behavior before it seriously interferes with the group's cohesion. Listed here are five categories of disruptive behavior as described by Bradford (1976) and expanded by these authors.

- Blocking—involves interruption of the group process by shifting the focus of attention from the issue to the blocker. Five kinds of blocking are anger, aggression, changing the topic of conversation, unconstructively arguing, and disagreeing without accepting compromise. These behaviors may be done either consciously or unintentionally, frequently in a stubborn or resistant way, as a result of fear, anxiety, or hostility.
- Power seeking—usually occurs between the leader and another individual or subgroup of individuals. May be done directly to gain authority or indirectly to form a protective coalition of a few members who individually are threatened by the group process. Power seeking tends to isolate the group members while it spotlights the interaction of a few. It can be particularly threatening to an inexperienced leader.
- Recognition seeking—occurs when a member draws undue attention toward him- or herself by displaying inappropriate or annoying behavior. The person frequently seems to talk for the sake of talking without adding any new ideas or insights to the discussion. Many times this includes a story or anecdote using him- or herself as the star. A recognition seeker may periodically disengage from the group, only to return and request attention. In some situations, behaviors may be unusual or extreme and offensive to the group.
- Dominating—includes behaviors that consume group time and monopolize the communication, such as endless speeches, definitive pronouncements, and lobbying for a favorite cause. This deprives other members of time to participate. Unlike power seekers, who want authority, and recognition seekers, who need personal attention, dominators simply prevent other, less assertive members from sharing. Dominators may actually feel inferior to others, and their behavior is an attempt to be involved. It is helpful to involve these members in a task they are quite capable of doing, thus enhancing their security. Give positive reinforcement and encourage others to be patient.
- Clowning—although occasional use of humor can ease the seriousness and tenseness of any group, persistent joking and laughing can be distracting. It indicates a lack of involvement in the group and may represent insecurity and lack of confidence in oneself. Frequently, a clowning member needs positive reinforcement, support, and empathy from others.

Most of these dysfunctional behaviors can best be handled by the skillful use of verbal feedback. Most frequently, disruptive members are behaving as they do unintentionally and innocently. A warm, friendly, sensitive person can point out behaviors without being threatening or punitive. By objectively stating exactly what is occurring and the effect it has on the group, you can enhance the member's self-awareness. It is helpful to offer alternative behaviors and focus the discussion on the positive rather than the negative. There may be times when constructive confrontation is appropriate in the presence of the entire group. One must carefully consider the effects that confrontation may have on an individual member and act accordingly. Disruptive behavior should be dealt with as early as possible, lest it get out of hand and cause irreversible anger and hostility among the group members. This anger and frustration can potentially be redirected toward a leader who is perceived as not resolving the problem and as responsible for doing so (Sampson & Marthas, 1977, p. 252).

WHAT IS LEADERSHIP?

All groups develop a leadership style. Styles can be described as authoritarian, democratic, or laissez-faire. Authoritarian leadership specifically puts someone in charge to make decisions and plans and to resolve differences. It gives the responsibility clearly to one person who has the final say.

Members in democratic groups mutually develop and share responsibilities. Authority is delegated as members' capabilities emerge. The democratic leader devotes attention to facilitating the members' growth and participation.

The least active leader is one with a laissez-faire style. He or she believes that things will happen on their own and so assumes a very passive, nondecisive role. This leader is frequently visible in presence only.

It is obvious that membership and participation in each type of group is very different. Lippett and White (1953) studied these differences, with some interesting findings. They concluded that groups with authoritarian leadership were quite efficient and very dependent on the leader. When the leader withdrew, group effectiveness diminished, and members became confused as to what to do. The least productive groups studied were those with a laissez-faire leadership style. Members had little guidance and direction, resulting in frustration, discontent, and boredom. Not surprisingly, perhaps, the most productive groups in these experiments were the democratic ones. These members were the friendliest most creative and involved. They had strong interest, motivation, and energy.

It can be summarized that most professional helpers operate in a framework that combines authoritarian and democratic characteristics. It is important for a leader to recognize the type of climate created.

Sometimes groups choose to have more than one leader. This is done either by co-leadership or rotating leadership. There are some obvious disadvantages, though, and groups must be sensitive to them. Co-leaders may not complement each other and, thus, cause tenseness and divisiveness in the group. When a rotating leadership role is chosen, there is little opportunity for a member to feel a sense of role security and authority. Individual guidance and nurturing are minimal. Some group members may not be effective as leaders.

Removing the burden of leadership from one individual has many advantages, however, especially if the leader is overwhelmed. Co-leadership allows functions to be divided and shared. One leader, for instance, may devote attention to the task function aimed at accomplishing the group purpose. Simultaneously, the other leader can direct attention to the feelings of the individual members, attempting to enhance the participation of each.

Rotating the leadership role helps each member gain an appreciation for this responsibility. It can enhance members' subsequent cooperation with the leader. Changing leaders allows a diversity of strengths to emerge, enhancing the chances that all of the task and maintenance functions will be addressed.

The role of an effective leader is a complex one, requiring a great deal of understanding and strengthened by each leadership experience. There is no formula for being a successful leader, but there are certain assumptions one should hold:

1. Leadership is shared by the membership rather than always assumed by one individual. Shared leadership:

   > happens when any intervention by the leader or a group member moves the group forward toward three goals: the accomplishment of the task, the resolution of internal group problems, and the ability of the members to work together effectively as a group. (Bradford, 1976, p. 10)

   Group-centered leadership fosters cohesion and satisfaction, but it takes time and patience. One of the most difficult challenges for any group leader is simply to be a catalyst. This requires a deep understanding of group dynamics, sensitive communication skills, and a strong self-concept.

2. Leadership involves therapeutic communication skills and necessitates keen observation and perceptive, sensitive listening. Attention to verbal and nonverbal cues, overt and covert behaviors, as well as the feelings and emotions of members, is a necessity. Empathy and acceptance of others is crucial. If the leader is unable to express him- or herself clearly and help others to do the same, then the entire communication process is confused. Multidirectional participation should be encouraged and diversity of opinion permitted.

3. Leadership involves promoting growth both of the group and of its members. A leader accepts responsibility for helping a group achieve its goals. The leader also facilitates the growth of individuals. A supportive environment that diminishes the sense of risk and competition, encourages trust and cooperation, and expands self-awareness is optimal. A successful leader realizes that individuals and groups are never static, but always internally dynamic. Consequently, the leader supports change and directly, yet calmly, confronts conflicts and problems as they arise, using a systematic method of problem management.

Throughout the group process, the leader encourages participation and involvement of all members.

GROUPS AS A MODEL OF HELPING

To those of us in the helping professions, groups have a special meaning. For teachers and sociologists, they are the primary vehicle of the profession. In psychology, nursing, and occupational therapy they provide an alternative way of enhancing a client's health and adaptation. Groups enable us to help a greater number of people within a given period of time. Additionally, they can enhance the client's growth and self-esteem by demonstrating that there are people who are supportive and caring and who may be experiencing similar feelings. They provide a sense of belonging and security at a time of emotional vulnerability.

Leading successful groups is a challenge and an art. While special skills can be learned and experience can be gained, sensitivity and concern cannot. They must be genuine and given freely. The helping professional preparing for tomorrow's action must have a firm foundation in group theory and dynamics. This will enable the professional to become creatively involved with clients seeking help.

IMPORTANT REMINDERS

1. The concept of group is basic to the helping professions, just as it is basic to life.
2. Effective, mature groups are united toward a purpose and, in the process of accomplishing their objectives, enhance growth of the individual as well as the group.
3. Effective groups are dependent upon responsible members who support the group's structure, facilitate the group process, and share the group's functions.
4. The skills needed to lead a group can be learned, but they alone cannot assure success. Sensitivity, perception, and genuine concern are primary components of helping.
5. The ultimate goal of successful group leadership—and of helping professions—is to create and/or facilitate client independence.

REFERENCES

Benne, K., & Sheats, P. (1948, Spring). Functional roles of group members. In L. P. Bradford and J. R. French Jr. (Eds.), *The Journal of Social Issues*, 4(2).
Bernstein, S. (1973). *Explorations in group work*. Boston: Milford House.

Bradford, L. (1976). *Making meetings work*. La Jolla, Calif.: University Association.

Coffey, H. S. (1966). Group psychotherapy. In J. A. Berg & L. A. Pennington (Eds.), *Introduction to clinical psychology*. New York: Ronald Press.

Combs, A., Avila, D., & Purkey, W. (1971). *Helping relationships—basic concepts for the helping professions*. Boston: Allyn & Bacon.

Gerrard, B., Boniface, W., & Love, B. (1980). *Interpersonal skills for health professionals*. Reston, Va.: Reston Publishing.

Lacoursiere, R. B. (1980). *The life cycle of groups*. New York: Human Sciences Press.

Leavitt, H. J. (1958). Some effects of certain communication patterns on group performance. In E. E. Maccoby, T. M. Newcomb, & E. L. Hartley (Eds.), *Readings in social psychology* (3rd ed.). New York: Holt, Rinehart, & Winston.

Lippett, R., & White, R. (1953). Leader behavior and member reaction in three social climates. In D. Cartwright & A. Zander (Eds.), *Group dynamics*. Evanston, Ill.: Row Peterson.

Loomis, M. E. (1979). *Group process for nurses*. St. Louis: C. V. Mosby.

Marram, G. (1978). *The group approach in nursing practice*. St. Louis: C. V. Mosby.

McCann-Flynn, J. B., & Heffron, P. (1984). *Nursing from concept to practice*. Bowie, Md.: Robert Brady.

Moreno, J. L. (1951). *Sociometry, experimental method and the science of society*. Beacon, N.Y.: Beacon House.

Sampson, E., & Marthas, M. (1977). *Group process for the health professions*. New York: Wiley.

Semrad, E., & Arsenian, J. (1975). The use of group processes in teaching group dynamics. *American Journal of Psychiatry, 108*, 258–363.

Smith, S. L. (1951). Communication patterns and the adaptabilty of task-oriented groups: An experimental study. In D. Lerner & H. Lasswell (Eds.), *The policy sciences: Recent developments in scope and method*. Stanford, Calif.: Stanford University Press.

Vinter, R. (Ed.). (1967). *Readings in group work practice*. Ann Arbor; Mich.: Campus Publishers.

Yalon, I., & Terrazas, F. (1968). *Group therapy with chronic psychiatric patients*. Unpublished manuscript, Modesto Hospital, Modesto, Calif.

No matter what kind of trouble a man has, he is sure to prefer some other kind.

Anonymous

Threat

Upon completion of the following reading and suggested exercises, the student will be able to:

1. Define the concepts of threat, anxiety, fear, and stress.
2. Identify biophysical, psychosocial, and cognitive behaviors that occur when threat impinges upon a person's self-esteem and identity.
3. Discuss how threat can promote growth.
4. Recognize problem solving as a necessary component in adapting to threatening situations.
5. Identify intervention techniques that can be used to help clients adapt effectively to threatening situations.

RESPONSES TO THREAT: ANXIETY, STRESS, AND FEAR

*Fear**

Barnabus Browning
Was scared of drowning,
So he never would swim
Or get into a boat
Or take a bath
Or cross a moat.
He just sat day and night

With his door locked tight
And the windows nailed down,
Shaking with fear
That a wave might appear,
And cried so many tears
That they filled up the room
And he drowned.

---

*From *A Light in the Attic; Poems and Drawings* by Shel Silverstein. Copyright © 1981 by Snake Eye Music, Inc. By permission of Harper & Row, Publishers, Inc.

We would like to acknowledge the contributions of Marylee Evans who wrote this chapter in the first edition of *Basic Concepts of Helping*.

Barnabus Browning's plight is really quite devastating. His response to threat is fear—overwhelming fear; poor Barnabus is never to overcome this fear, as he inevitably succumbs to it. As helpers, you will meet clients that have equally devastating plights, and your ability to respond appropriately is extremely important. As with all helping skills, your response is contingent upon your understanding of the concept of threat and its responses: anxiety, fear, and stress.

Anxiety . . . fear . . . stress . . . common words to all of us. Our perceptions, feelings, and thoughts associated with these, however, may not be so similar. It is rare that any two people are affected by a situation in exactly the same way. Since people are unique and bring different life experiences to a situation, their perceptions frequently differ. It is a person's perception of the events that influences the intensity of response. Even in the same person, the response to two similar situations may differ at various times throughout life. Consider the relationship of perception and threat in the following example:

> Kathy Light is a 30-year-old mother of two boys, Albert, 3, and Michael, 1. Michael was hospitalized when he was 8 months old for a severe upper respiratory tract infection. Thus, when he becomes ill, Kathy watches him very carefully, as she is afraid that he might have to be hospitalized again.
>
> One Tuesday Kathy becomes alarmed when she notices that Michael is having some difficulty breathing. After observing him for a couple of hours, she notes he has developed an obviously loud wheeze.
>
> At once she takes him to their pediatrician who, after thoroughly examining him, prescribes several medications and home treatments in an effort to cure what was diagnosed as bronchial asthma.
>
> Later that evening, Kathy becomes vividly apprehensive when Michael's breathing becomes markedly distressed. She calls the pediatrician, who suggests that she bring Michael to St. John's Hospital immediately. Kathy's heart pounds all the way to the hospital, not only at the sound of Michael's continual wheezing, but at the very thought that he might have to be hospitalized. Myriads of questions race through her mind. "Have I done something negligent as a mother to make him wheeze this way? Will he have to have injections? Will they have to perform other painful treatments? Will his wheezing become worse when he is left alone? Will he be all right? Could he—oh no—die?"

Kathy is obviously feeling threatened. Sundeen defines threat "as an anticipation of harm" (Sundeen, Stuart, Rankin, & Cohen, 1985, p. 208). Kathy really does not know what will happen to Michael when he enters the hospital. Because of previous experiences she is anticipating that all hospitalizations are unpleasant. She has an uneasy, uncomfortable feeling—the same feeling many of you have before a big exam. The first time Michael entered the hospital Kathy felt relieved; she did not anticipate anything harmful happening. This time she relates to a previous experience in which she remembers how Michael cried when she left to go home and how upset he became when given injections. It is important to realize that an actual threat need not be involved; a mere suggestion can create the same kind of response. Two weeks before this incident, Kathy took Michael to the doctor's office for a routine checkup. The doctor casually mentioned that Michael might need to be hospitalized again if he developed any more breathing problems. Although there were no apparent problems at the time, Kathy remembers having many of the same uncomfortable feelings that day as she does now.

Threatening stimuli continually bombard us daily. Kathy, like all of us, is constantly battling with potential threats to herself and others for whom she cares. For example, as a mother she continually deals with the fact that Michael may fall out of his crib or swallow a small object. These situations do not stimulate the same intensity of feeling that Michael's pending hospitalization does because Kathy's appraisal process distinguishes the two. It is important to note that threats are brought about by cognitive processes involving perceptions, learning, memory, judgment, and thought. It is these same· processes that enable us to appraise a potentially threatening situation.

In Kathy's situation, time and experience has enabled her to cope with some daily threats. She has developed behaviors that diminish the probability of these threats becoming harmful, i.e., vacuuming and picking up small objects each morning to keep them away from the hands and mouths of her children. She can cope with these because they are known and of low intensity. Also, she has a great deal of control over the home situation.

Michael's pending hospitalization, on the other hand, recalls unpleasant memories, is of high probability and intensity, and leaves her with little control. The situation and its outcome are less known and less tangible.

Thus, there is a cognitive process of appraisal occurring with potentially threatening stimuli:

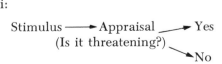

$$\text{Stimulus} \longrightarrow \text{Appraisal} \longrightarrow \text{Yes}$$
$$\text{(Is it threatening?)} \searrow \text{No}$$

Lazarus (1966) concludes that the degree of threat depends upon its amount, imminence, and probability. Stimuli are further identified as threatening or nonthreatening, depending upon the person's reaction to them. In other words, with the appraisal process, we are able to evaluate potentially threatening stimuli (Fig. 4–1). Some situations will be determined to be highly threatening (Michael's hospitalization) and others we will be capable of diminishing (the threat of Michael swallowing a small object). Consider the next example, in which it is clear that similar stimuli can be interpreted differently by individuals:

> Candy decides not to live in her college's dorm. She sets up housekeeping with one of her girlfriends, Joni, in a rural area outside of the university. Joni, who comes from a large city, is extremely careful to ensure each door and window has one or more working locks. Candy, who has a black belt in karate, thinks Joni is silly. She does not see unlocked doors and windows as a danger and dis-

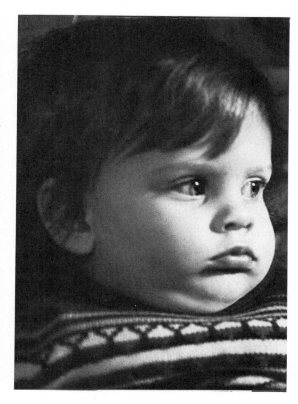

Figure 4-1. This toddler appears to be contemplating a threatening situation. Note that his pupils are large and his facial expression fixed and tense. *(Photo credit to Steve DeRosa.)*

misses Joni's concern. To Candy this is a weak threat and to Joni a very strong threat.

According to Peplau (1963) threats may be toward one's biological integrity or toward one's self-esteem and identity. In order to assess these threats, the helper must understand that the threat to one's self-integrity is usually associated with three underlying factors: (1) helplessness, (2) isolation, and (3) insecurity.

Let us examine these to determine how they relate to threatening events.

Michael, Kathy's 1-year-old son who is hospitalized, is threatened biologically because of his inability to control his breathing. He is also feeling a threat to his security because Mommy, a significant person in his life, has left him in the hospital. At this moment, he is in a helpless situation; there is nothing he can do to overcome his environment or physical condition.

Michael is left alone confined to a crib and surrounded by an oxygen tent. For safety reasons, he is restrained with a chest binder. His mother has left, and there is no one in the room with whom he has direct contact. Michael is feeling isolated—totally alone.

Michael begins to regress in his new environment. He was just about weaned from a bottle and had just begun to walk before entering the hospital. However, in the hospital he has not attempted to walk, wanting to be carried everywhere, and he has screamed at night until given a bottle. Michael is feeling very insecure in this new environment, and because he is unable to adapt to the situation at his normal developmental level, he finds that regressing to previous behaviors helps him gain some security.

As a helper assessing a client's behavior, you must recognize that helplessness, insecurity, isolation, and interruption in biological integrity all contribute to the creation of a sense of being threatened. These may be present individually or in combination. The client's feelings are not always easily identifiable, and it is important throughout your relationship to continually assess that which you feel may be threatening.

Often much of the threatening feeling that a client experiences can be minimized. Once the helper is able to identify those stimuli that the client finds threatening, a plan can be devised to minimize or eliminate them. Certain threats, however, are imminent and impossible to minimize. Clients need help learning how to cope with these annoying threats. Note how Harry Rooney, aged 73, learns to cope with his wife, Sally's, diagnosis of terminal cancer:

After 50 years of a blissful marriage, Harry is initially devastated by the news of his wife's illness. "What if she dies now—how will I manage? Can I go on?" asks Harry.

The nursing staff spends a long time helping Harry, answering his questions, and encouraging him to verbalize feelings. After doing this, they help Harry and his wife by encouraging them to take one day at a time. Eventually, Harry and Sally work out funeral arrangements together and made plans for Harry's future living arrangements. The threat of death does not leave—it is inevitable. Harry is able, however, to alter his response and effectively work on minimizing the threat. By the time Sally dies, Harry has begun to feel he can cope effectively.

We have seen that potentially threatening stimuli cause a normal process to occur in all of us. This happens many times a day, resulting in varied responses depending upon one's level of adaptation and perception of the situation. Generally speaking, people respond to threat with feelings of anxiety, fear, or stress. Most often people are able to cope successfully and problem solve effectively.

"When abilities and resources are wanting, the person . . . usually seeks help from others to compensate for the temporary inability to deal constructively with life's stressors (threats). This help is crisis intervention" (Hoff, 1984, p. 79). It is derived from either professional or social helping relationships. When the help of professionals is sought, "there is need to assess in detail the parameters of the individual's vulnerability" (Hoff, 1984, p. 79). One must understand the biophysical, psychosocial, and cognitive responses. It should be noted that "it is not the events of our lives that activate crisis. Crisis occurs when our interpretation of these events, our coping ability, and the limitation of our social resources lead to [threat] so severe that we cannot find relief" (Hoff, 1984, p. 5). While anxiety, fear, and stress responses are similar in many ways, there are some significant differences that influence the helper's assessment and subsequent care.

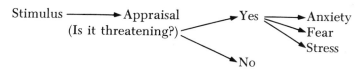

Let us first define anxiety, fear, and stress and then explore ways of discussing clients' responses and enhancing adaptation.

Anxiety

"Anxiety is probably the most common and universal behavioral response to any threat, real or imagined" (Infante, 1982, p. 237). It is an emotional state that results when one's biological integrity or self-esteem is threatened. It is characterized by subjective feelings of uneasiness, worry, apprehension, nervousness, and a sense of dread and foreboding. As such, it is a response to the threat of future danger from something unknown and vague. It should be emphasized that anxiety results from one's perception of threat. Regardless of whether the threat is real or imagined, the anxious, uncomfortable feeling occurs. Anxiety frequently happens, not because threats are overwhelming, but because they are new and an inadequate defense system is unprepared to handle them. Because anxiety "is provoked by the unknown, it precedes all new experiences, such as entering school, starting a new job, or giving birth to a child" (Stuart & Sundeen, 1983, p. 207). In Kathy's first experience with Michael's hospitalization, she is unable to adequately cope with and resolve the crisis, not because it was overwhelming, but because she has never been in the situation. Since Kathy has no former experiences of this nature, she has never had to develop coping patterns for this type of situation and, therefore, had no reserve upon which to call. Usually an individual such as Michael or Kathy, with limited past experiences and resources, who encounters a threatening new experience will have a fair amount of anxiety. Their experiential backgrounds have not prepared them to handle the situation.

Anxiety is common to all of us and a testament to our humanness (Portnoy, 1959). It is normal, healthy, and necessary. By eliciting our "fight-or-flight" response, anxiety motivates us to make plans and take action, acquire new skills and behaviors, and learn to cope with new situations. For example, it is frequently the anxiety you feel before an exam that heightens your awareness and motivates you to study. Without a bit of anxiety you might not be nearly so well prepared!

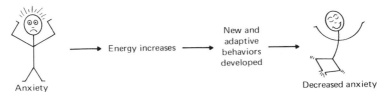

Figure 4-2. Growth-producing experience.

Life experiences can present anxious times that are predictable. For example, as we grow and confront developmental transition stages in life such as adolescence and senescence, there is a natural change in role, body image, and attitude toward oneself and the world that naturally heightens anxiety (Hoff, 1984). With each successful adaptation, we become better prepared to cope with our next new experience. We become more experienced with adapting our old ways and developing new behaviors and skills.

Anxiety is frequently classified according to degree as mild, moderate, or severe. Almost everyone experiences mild anxiety during the course of a day, whereas people in crisis usually have a severe degree of anxiety. For some people severe anxiety becomes chronic or continual.

Mild anxiety heightens one's senses, increasing attentiveness, perception, and cognitive effectiveness. One is capable of learning new skills and ideas and has increased energy and motivation to do so. Even though there is tension, adaptation potential is high and the experience is growth-producing. Recalling your first job interview, the beginning of a new semester, or getting ready for a much desired date will remind you how it feels to be mildly anxious. It is not necessarily negative (Fig. 4-2).

With moderate anxiety one's overall effectiveness begins to diminish. As tension increases, the ability to adapt independently decreases. Direction and support are needed for effective problem solving and learning to occur. "The person becomes consumed by anxiety and is less able to focus on the realities of the situation and productively channel energies. . . . Perceptual field narrows" (Grace & Camilleri, 1981, p. 107). While there are some people who can effectively function while moderately anxious, most cannot. Crying, anger, irritability, forgetfulness, and demanding behavior might be expected.

> Jim Rodes is one of three finalists waiting to hear whether he has been selected for a position at the local bank. He describes himself as excited and hopeful, but uneasy. He is having difficulty sleeping, and his appetite has diminished. While his energy level is high, he cannot seem to concentrate at work. His wife is upset because he is neglecting his daily home responsibilities and does not seem to care about their daughter's recent problems at school.

As anxiety continues to mount, one's usual responses are no longer effective, and crisis occurs. With severe anxiety, one's perception is distorted,

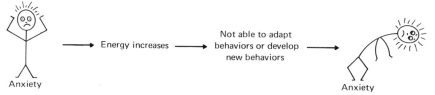

Figure 4-3. Growth-inhibiting experience.

memory and reasoning are altered, and attention and ability to learn are impaired (Fig. 4–3). This "state of anguish and resulting confusion can alter a person's ability to make decisions and solve problems, the very skills needed during a crisis . . . the individual's already heightened state of anxiety increases" (Hoff, 1984, p. 81). But Hoff reminds us that:

> The distorted perceptual process observed in crisis states should not be confused with mental illness, in which a person's usual pattern of thinking is disturbed. In a crisis state, the disturbance arises from and is part of the crisis experience. There is a rapid return to normal perception once the crisis is resolved. (Hoff, 1984, p. 81)

The extreme result of severe anxiety may be panic or total incapacitation.

> Isadora Jenssen, a chemist, panicked when her husband, Marc, began to choke on a piece of meat. Someone in the room told her to call the rescue squad. She cried, "I don't know how!"

Stress

Stress is a reaction to any stimulus, known or unknown, that causes us to change in order to maintain homeostasis. Thus, it occurs constantly in living things. It is inevitable and not to be avoided. Many of the great achievements of mankind have occurred as a result of stress. Stress can be growth-producing. When stress mounts, however, it can become a negative force and interferes with high-level adaptation. In those situations, one's goal is to minimize its effects and manage to cope successfully with it. Hans Selye, one of the leading researchers of stress, concluded that:

> Anything that causes stress endangers life, unless it is met by adequate adaptive responses; conversely, anything that endangers life causes stress and adaptive responses. Adaptability and resistance to stress are fundamental prerequisites for life, and every vital organ and function participates in them. (Selye, 1956, p. 467)

It is generally accepted that stress is always present within a person and is intensified when there is a change, stressor, or threat with which one must cope (Byrne & Thompson, 1978). This threat may be from pleasant or unpleasant experiences in the internal or external environment. Thus, jogging 5 miles in the morning, although enjoyable, creates much physical stress.

Stress demands a holistic—physical, psychological, and cognitive—response, either overtly or covertly. "How one reacts to stress is an individual matter. It would depend on how one perceives the threat . . . the degree of change caused by it, and the individual's ability to adapt" (McCann-Flynn & Heffron, 1984, p. 515). Like anxiety, stress in mild amounts is necessary for development, since it serves as a motivating factor to increase one's functioning and productivity. It is necessary for survival and life. In fact, the absence of stress means stagnation and death. Even during the sleep process, the body functions under a degree of stress to maintain vital functions.

When stress occurs briefly and is of short duration, it is acute and probably has few or no long-term negative effects on the individual. Insidious stress, however, may last years and is believed to have long-term cumulative effects, including disease (Landry, 1977, p. 311). Recently much public attention has been given to the effects of chronic stress and ways in which one can reduce it in daily living. It is believed that becoming familiar with one's own reaction to stress and seeking emotional and physical diversions can be beneficial. Emphasis has been placed on maintaining healthy practices and keeping physically fit.

Fear

The emotional outcome of a threatening situation also can be fear—the feeling of dread and apprehension in response to an external source that is clearly identifiable and definable.

> You have an 89 average in chemistry and have studied for 2 weeks for the final exam. Just before you take the exam, you have an uneasy feeling, which you cannot explain. You know you have a passing average and have done your best to prepare well. This is anxiety. If, however, you have a 56 average in chemistry and have not studied well for the final exam, you may be fearful that you will fail the course. The key characteristic of fear is that it is directed at "a specific source or object which the person can identify and describe" (Stuart & Sundeen, 1983, p. 207).

In this example the fear is realistic; you may indeed fail the course. But sometimes fears are unjustifiable and irrational. In such cases it is important for helpers to remember that it is the client's perception of fear that is significant. Like stress and anxiety, fears may be described as mild, moderate, or severe.

ADAPTATIONS TO THREAT: BIOPHYSICAL, COGNITIVE, AND PSYCHOSOCIAL

We have learned that when one is confronted with a stimulus appraised as being threatening, the responses are anxiety, fear, and/or stress (Fig. 4–4). The behaviors and feelings that occur with anxiety, fear, and stress can be observed and measured. Accurate assessment of these becomes crucial when providing care to clients. For if we are to help clients effectively, we must have accurate data and understanding of their problems. Our interventions and care are dependent upon accurate diagnosis.

Assessment includes the observation of objective data, called *signs*, and the eliciting of subjective feelings from the client, called *symptoms*. It includes the biophysical, psychosocial, and cognitive modes.

Biophysical Adaptation

Anxiety, fear, and stress manifest themselves in similar ways. There are a variety of behaviors that may occur. Those that are objective and can be observed are such things as perspiring, shaking, deep and rapid breathing, a palpitating

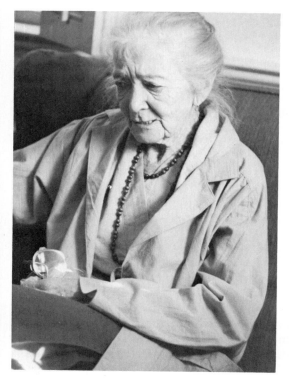

Figure 4-4. Which response to threat do you think this women is experiencing? *(Photo credit to Peggy Haggerty.)*

heartbeat, and dilated pupils. There are other manifestations that are less obvious and can only be obtained by laboratory testing. Some examples of these would be an elevated secretion of catecholamines or an elevated blood pressure. The eliciting of subjective data is equally important, but may take more time. Therapeutic communication skills facilitate such assessment. Some subjective biophysical feelings that may be reported by a person are "butterfly" stomach, uneasiness, stage fright, a sensation of needing to urinate, or a scratchy throat. Helpers cannot always identify these physical responses within the client. Often the client may tell you of feelings—being particularly vague about the physical origins of the complaints but certain that something within is not right. Since you, as the helper, have no way of observing these uneasy feelings, you must regard what the client says with close scrutiny. To evaluate behavior purely on the objective behaviors is to limit your potential for helping. The effects of objective and subjective behaviors upon physiological functioning are dependent upon their intensity. It is important to remember that when people move from mild to severe levels of anxiety, fear, and stress, they expend more energy, adapt less effectively, and require more assistance.

A physiological response to threat activates both divisions of the autonomic nervous system, the sympathetic nervous system predominantly and the parasympathetic nervous system selectively, depending on the circumstances. The sympathetic nervous system prepares a person for confrontation or a hasty flight.

> For example, consider Patty, who looks up at the suddenly yellow sky and screams when she sees a dark funneling tornado heading her way. Physiologically, at this instant, her cerebral cortex perceives and interprets the stimulus as threatening and sends this message to the hypothalamus. Impulses are then sent to the skeletal muscles for the "fight-or-flight" response. Simultaneously, the autonomic nervous system receives messages from the cerebral cortex to innervate the visceral organs. As a result of this, Patty's heart beats faster, she breathes harder, and because certain blood vessels constrict, her face becomes pale and her blood pressure becomes elevated. She also is more alert, and her problem-solving ability has been increased. She is now ready to respond to the situation. Not thinking about her own safety, she starts looking for her daughter so she can shelter her from the tornado.

Since the sympathetic and parasympathetic nerve fibers are so close together, the latter may accidentally be stimulated when the sympathetic nervous system responds. Consequently, some behaviors occur that are the opposite of those behaviors stimulated by the sympathetic nervous system. For example, when Patty frantically looks for her daughter, who is nowhere to be found, she hurriedly looks up in the sky and notices the funnel is even closer now. She panics as she thinks she may not find her daughter in time. As a result, her pupils may constrict rather than dilate, she may feel nauseated and think she is going to vomit, and her blood pressure may drop. Normally, the parasympathetic nervous system is known to be more active during restful periods than during stressful times. It concentrates mainly on internal maintenance of the individual without concern for external problems. Therefore, digestion, excretion, and blood circulation, as well as other ordinary day-to-day maintenance activities, are its primary function and concern.

The endocrine system also plays a major role in biophysical adaptation to anxiety, fear, and stress. Although the response from the endocrine system takes longer to be initiated, its effects usually are more lasting than those of the autonomic nervous system. Alerted by the hypothalamus, the posterior pituitary gland secretes antidiuretic hormone (ADH), which helps the body retain fluid, thereby increasing the circulating blood volume and increasing the blood pressure. At this same time, the anterior pituitary gland secretes adrenocorticotrophic hormone (ACTH) in addition to other hormones. Of these, ACTH has the greatest effect and stimulates the adrenal cortex to secrete a variety of cortical steroid hormones. These help the body retain sodium (Na^+), which in turn retains water. This builds up blood volume and increases blood pressure. In addition, these hormones increase blood sugar to give the individual more energy to respond to the threat.

When the nervous system and endocrine system respond, the result is a systematic or whole response of the individual. Sometimes our body responds locally, however. This usually is necessary when there is a specific stress from within our body. In his pioneering work with stress, Hans Selye (1956) identified and described two types of stress reactions. The first of these is the Local Adaptative Syndrome (LAS), occurring within a person's body to limit the spread of the particular threat. Note the following example:

> Donna is a 30-year-old housewife and teacher. She is in the process of helping her husband remodel their home. Early one morning, she carelessly walks around barefoot and steps on a sharp piece of wood. Although she feels a splinter of wood in her foot, she is unable to remove it using her own home remedies. For the next couple of days she "favors" the foot with the splinter, saying it probably hurts because she stepped on a sharp object. By the third day she begins to note that the portion of her foot that touched the sharp object is reddened and swollen, as well as painful. She decides to see a doctor immediately, as she is afraid the area is infected and the infection might spread.

Fortunately, Donna has noted this infection and decided to take care of it while it is in its localized state. The splinter as a foreign object in her foot has caused white blood cells to come to the area in an attempt to repair the damage. At this point, the white blood cells have acted as a barrier preventing spread of the infection, therefore limiting the effect of the microbes causing the infection. This barrier is known as a "walling-off" process and is characteristic of LAS.

If Donna had chosen not to seek medical attention at this time, her entire foot and leg might have become involved. If the infection had spread, she would have noticed that her entire body—not just one specific area in her foot—felt uncomfortable. This would be an example of the second stress reaction Selye identified—the General Adaptative Syndrome (GAS). The GAS is characterized by the stages of alarm, resistance, and exhaustion.

The alarm stage occurs when the body is alerted to danger. At this point a person recognizes that there is some type of threat to physical integrity. In Donna's case, she began to identify this threat when she "favored" her foot. The threat became increasingly worse as she noted more pain, swelling, and redness in her foot. The body reacts in a uniquely biophysical sense by alerting us to impending danger. In this case, luckily, the forewarning arrived early enough and no permanent harm was done. As her foot became more painful, Donna's concern about a possible infection increased. Therefore, she began to think about alternatives other than "favoring her foot."

The stage of resistance is the body's way of adapting through internal responses that stimulate defense, mobilization, or action to regain equilibrium. Biophysically, this is in terms of tissue defense where protective mechanisms are stimulated. For example, white blood cells come to injured tissue with a specified purpose of ingesting foreign debris and microorganism, thus destroying the infection. Applying antibiotic cream would have been one way for Donna to promote the resistance stage and attempt to prevent tissue surrender.

The stage of exhaustion occurs when the person is not able to cope with or adapt to the threats as they are perceived. This occurs when previous adaptations have failed. Individuals at this level may seek help because it is obvious to them that they have a problem. The physical stress has become so overwhelming that the client's normal physiological adaptive mechanisms no longer function effectively.

Now let us think about biophysical response in a more personal way. How do you react when you become anxious, afraid, or are in a stressful situation? Think about the biophysical responses you experienced the last time you were in a threatening situation. Do cotton mouth, shaky knees, increased perspiration, heart palpitations, muscle tension, increased need to urinate, goose pimples, or stuttering sound familiar? Personal awareness of your own pattern of response and coping is necessary to attain professional maturity. Try to identify your assets as well as your limitations in functioning, especially in the area of interpersonal relationships. Through increased self-awareness, you will be able to build on your assets and decrease those limiting qualities that are a hindrance to you now. This will help you to become a more effective and empathetic helper.

Cognitive Adaptation

A person cognitively responds to threat by thinking about the situation. Mildly threatening situations enhance thinking by heightening awareness, concentrating attention, and sparking motivation. Usually one's perception of events is clear and problem-solving abilities are enhanced. As the threat increases, more assistance, support, and direction are needed, but with help, learning and decision making are still realistic expectations. When moderately threatened, one's perception of events may become clouded or skewed. The threatening stimuli may overwhelm functioning temporarily.

Peggy has been studying all week for her biology exam. Biology is her major, and she really wants to do well in the course. She is experiencing some anxiety and stress, but not enough to hinder her performance on the exam. In fact, her anxiety is motivating Peggy to study harder.

Joan is also studying for the biology exam. Since it is her major, she would like to receive a high grade in the course. She also has a history exam on that day, and a final lab report due the next day for her chemistry class. Joan has had an argument with her roommate and has not been able to study comfortably in her room. Joan is an extremely conscientious student. Although she has studied for the exam, when she is handed the test she panics and is unable to think clearly. The events of the past week and the demands of the immediate future seem to overpower her thinking ability. In effect, her mind has gone "blank."

With severe reactions to threat, cognitive processes are markedly altered. Perception becomes distorted; objective thinking and adaptive efficiency are unattainable. Decision making and learning may be overwhelmingly difficult or impossible.

Researchers have investigated the influences of anxiety on learning, concept formation, and academic achievement. In a number of studies Spielberger (1966) found that high-anxiety students performed poorly on difficult tests in comparison with low-anxiety students. He showed that academic failure occurred nearly four times more often with high-anxiety students than it did with low-anxiety students of the same aptitude.

People who are feeling threatened frequently seem caught in a maze of happenings they cannot fit together. The situation they find themselves in does not make sense. This state of confusion can alter their ability to think, make decisions, and solve problems. The very skills they need fail them. These disturbances in critical thinking and logic may increase already heightened states of anxiety, fear, or stress.

As a helper, it behooves you to understand your own cognitive responses to threat. How do you respond during professional crises? How clearly will you think when your patient has a cardiac arrest or the student you are teaching attempts suicide? Think about how you have reacted to anxiety, fear, or stress in the past. What happens to your ability to think, to problem solve, and to make decisions? It is important that you increase your self-awareness so as to understand your own cognitive responses. Remember, clients in crisis expect helpers to be calm, competent, and critical thinkers who can provide strength when they, the clients, are temporarily weak.

Psychosocial Adaptation

When a threat impinges upon a person's self-esteem and identity, a psychosocial adaptation occurs, which enables the person to maintain composure and stability. This has frequently been referred to as *defensive behavior*. Freud (1959) initially described defensive behavior as that which was initiated by the ego to avoid a threat.

A brief description and example of some of the more common defense mechanisms are given in Table 4–1. From time to time, all of us have used adaptive mechanisms to cope with threatening situations. Generally, people become comfortable utilizing certain specific mechanisms that work best for them, thus establishing styles or patterns of coping.

The use of defense mechanisms, however, is unconscious. Obviously, this must be so if their purpose is to conceal the threat from one's awareness. In other words, a person does not knowingly select and use a specific defense mechanism at will. Rather, one unconsciously selects certain behaviors to protect oneself from harm. It stands to reason that if a particular adaptive mechanism has worked successfully before, it will be used repeatedly as long as threat continues to be reduced. Thus, patterns of coping occur in people. The patterns of behavior originate in the early formative years of childhood when we are first exposed to anxiety-producing or stressful circumstances. If a certain mechanism is successful in reducing the fear, stress, or anxiety in a particular situation, it will be used again because we can reliably predict how the situation will turn out. The more the adaptive mechanism successfully reduces our discomfort, the more repeatedly it will be used. By the time we are adults, these adaptation patterns may become habitual and are often very hard to alter.

> Joshua Brent has been afraid of sleeping in the dark since early childhood. As a college student he knows he can no longer sleep with the hall light on, so he buys a small night light and finds it works quite well.

The use of psychological mechanisms often provide healthy alternatives to less healthy behaviors. For example, it is far better for a man to rip up a picture of a former lover than to batter her! (Sublimation!) While enabling us to respond in a healthier, more acceptable, and more productive fashion, defense mechanisms frequently buy time. Denial, for example, enables one to simply not deal with the full impact of a threatening situation until one is psychologically ready to do so.

As a helper, you may need to assist a client in recognizing the use of a defense mechanism. While generally they are healthy and helpful, defense mechanisms can inhibit effective problem solving and hinder personal growth. By helping a person understand how uncomfortable situations are handled, you may enable the person to change undesirable behaviors. Confronting a client with this type of reality may be a painful process for both of you. However, allowing the client to hide behind his or her defenses only puts a "halt" to progress in dealing with the threats in the environment. As a helper, you need to assist the client in gaining a realistic perspective about his or her reactions to stress, anxiety, and fear. Once the client gains insight into these reactions, you can help the client move in a forward direction. This will enhance high-level adaptation to future threats throughout life.

TABLE 4-1. COMMON DEFENSE MECHANISMS

Defense Mechanism	Example
Introjection The unconscious internalization of the qualities and values of another person or group so that they become a part of the self.	When Albert's kitty makes a mess of a stack of newspapers, he scolds the kitty just as his mommy does him.
Projection The opposite of introjection. The placing of one's own unacceptable feelings onto another person or object in an attempt to liberate the individual from any association with that which is unfavorable.	Susan willingly participates in a sexual relationship with Tom, and then tells people he forced her to do so.
Reaction Formation Occurs when one replaces an attitude, feeling, or behavior with an opposite attitude, feeling, or behavior.	Michael is the "ideal" patient. Kathy is scared to death but smiles very confidently.
Sublimation To unconsciously divert unacceptable instinctual drives such as sex and aggression into more personally and socially acceptable channels.	Jack takes out all of his anger by playing racquetball each week.
Denial Is the mind's way of unconsciously obscuring awareness and avoiding a disturbing reality situation, thought, need, feeling, etc.	Mary continually plans social outings with her frail and sickly grandmother even though they are never able to go.
Regression The return of specific aspects of the personality to former levels of development or earlier modes of behavior.	Michael has been successfully drinking from a cup at home but during his hospitalization refuses a cup and drinks from a bottle only. During this crisis, his mother, Kathy has been biting her nails and chain smoking. These are habits she stopped 2 years previously.
Identification A person's unconscious attempt to pattern him- or herself after another as that person is perceived to be.	You have been spending a lot of time with a certain colleague whom you respect. All of a sudden you note you are talking like that colleague— using many of the same expressions.
Repression Puts or restricts unpleasant thoughts, feelings, and events in the subconscious so that one is not consciously aware of them.	Mrs. Smith does not remember her husband hitting her.

(continued)

TABLE 4-1. (continued)

Defense Mechanism	Example
Dissociation Unconsciously separating one's emotions into separate compartments and thereby enabling the emotional significance to be detached from an idea or event.	Mr. Thompson reprimands his students for watching pornographic films at a party but stops on the way home from school to pick up some "girlie" magazines.
Compensation Occurs when an individual attempts to overemphasize or make up for a handicap, limitation, or some other deficiency that is either real or imagined. This mechanism can be both conscious and unconscious.	A man who has always regretted being small in stature works hard to become a strong and influential judge.
Rationalization The unconscious process whereby one attempts to justify thoughts, feelings, or behaviors that are unacceptable or not necessarily rational or logical. The individual avoids admitting the truth about a particular situation.	A nursing student is given a low grade because she gave poor care to her patients. She says this is because no one taught her how to give good care.
Undoing Performance of a specific act that is unconsciously considered the opposite of a previous unacceptable act in an attempt to neutralize the original act. In essence, the individual tries to undo an unpleasant situation.	When Michael spills his milk all over the Christmas cards Kathy has just finished addressing, she spanks him. Later, she spends extra time playing his favorite games and romping with him in the living room.

Sometimes, a defense mechanism may begin to control rather than protect the personality. Or, if it is overused, the effectiveness diminishes and the client's escape from reality becomes pathological. This person needs the assistance of a psychologist, psychiatric nurse, or psychiatrist.

As a helper, you need to be aware of your own use of adaptive mechanisms. Do you tend to avoid or run away from difficult situations, or do you remain with the situation and attempt to reduce or neutralize the threat? And how do you do this? Do you evaluate and analyze your reactions and coping styles in order to promote both personal and professional growth, or do you just forget about the threat so you will not have to deal with it? Before you are able to understand and deal with another's anxiety and stress, you must first know and understand your own.

IMPLICATIONS FOR THE HELPER

We have seen that anxiety, fear, and stress are all responses to threat in the internal and external environment. As such, they are healthy signals for us to adapt psychologically, cognitively, and biophysically. As long as a person is not overwhelmed by threat, his or her coping behavior will probably be successful. But it is frequently professional helpers who assist clients in adaptation. If done in a timely fashion, the anxiety-fear-stress cycle can be broken. Reinforcing positive coping behaviors in the client enhances wellness and supports independence.

Although it is relatively easy for the helper to point out strengths in the client's coping ability, sometimes it is necessary to point out weaknesses. An open willingness to confront the person directly with your observations can be very helpful. This will enable the person to begin to assume activities that will help maintain or regain integrity and self-esteem. Once the client reaches an awareness of these reactions to threatening stimuli, he or she is ready to begin investigating means of diminishing these responses. In doing so, the client will be better equipped physically, emotionally, and intellectually to solve future problems.

IMPORTANT REMINDERS

1. Unknown threats to one's biological integrity or self-esteem cause anxiety; known threats cause fear; and both cause stress.
2. Anxiety, fear, and stress are normal, inevitable parts of everyday living and are manifested in the biophysical, psychosocial, and cognitive modes.
3. Every person has patterns of adaptation developed as a result of previous life experiences.
4. That which constitutes anxiety, fear, and stress to one person may not do the same to another.
5. Mild to moderate levels of threat serve as motivational factors for a person, helping one to make appropriate plans and to take constructive action. As the degree of threat intensifies, the coping responses become less effective, and adaptation diminishes.

REFERENCES

Byrne, M. L., & Thompson, L. F. (1978). *Key concepts for the study and practice of nursing* (2nd ed.). St. Louis: C. V. Mosby.

Freud, S. (1959). [Inhibitions, symptoms, and anxiety.] In J. Stachery (trans.), *[Standard edition of the complete works of Sigmund Freud]* (Vol. 20). London: Hogarth Press. (Originally published, 1926.)

Grace, H., & Camilleri, D. (1981). *Mental health nursing: A socio-psychological approach* (2nd ed.). Dubuque, Iowa: Brown.

Hoff, L. A. (1984). *People in crisis: Understanding and helping* (2nd ed.). Menlo Park, Calif.: Addison-Wesley.

Infante, M. S. (Ed.). (1982). *Crisis theory: A framework for nursing practice.* Reston, Va.: Reston Publishing.

Landry, D. (1977). *Culture, disease, and healing: Studies in medical anthropology.* New York: Macmillan.

Lazarus, R. S. (1966). *Psychological stress and the coping process.* New York: McGraw-Hill.

McCann-Flynn, J. B., & Heffron, P. B. (1984). *Nursing from concept to practice.* Bowie, Md.: Robert Brady.

Peplau, H. (1963). A working definition of anxiety. In S. F. Burd & M. A. Marshall (Eds.). *Some clinical approaches to psychiatric nursing.* London: Macmillan.

Portnoy, I. (1959). Anxiety states. In S. Arieti (Ed.), *American handbook of psychiatry.* New York: Basic Books.

Selye, H. (1956). *The stress of life.* New York: McGraw-Hill.

Silverstein, S. (1981). *A light in the attic.* New York: Harper & Row.

Spielberger, C. D. (Ed.). (1966). *Anxiety and behavior.* New York: Academic Press.

Stuart, G., & Sundeen, S. (1983). *Principles and practice of psychiatric nursing.* St. Louis. C. V. Mosby.

Sundeen, S., Stuart, G., Rankin, E., & Cohen, S. (1985). *Nurse–client interaction* (3rd ed.). St. Louis. C. V. Mosby.

A stranger's kindness oft exceeds a friend's.

Thomas Middleton

5

Helping

Upon completion of the following reading and suggested exercises, the student will be able to:

1. Describe the historical evolution of professional helpers.
2. Identify four goals of professional helping.
3. Compare and contrast social and professional relationships.
4. Explain the progression of a helping relationship through the stages of trust formation, resistance, working phase, and termination.
5. Discuss the concept of trust and how one promotes it in a professional relationship.
6. Discuss the feelings that a client may have about entering into and participating in a professional helping relationship.
7. Describe the characteristics, feelings, and needs of a helping person.
8. Explore your potential as a professional helper.

We would like to acknowledge the contributions of Brenda Bissell, who wrote this chapter in the first edition of *Basic Concepts of Helping*.

I wish there were Someone
Who would hear confession:
Not a priest—I do not want to be told of my sins;
Not a mother—I do not want to give sorrow;
Not a friend—she would not know enough;
Not a lover—he would be too partial;
Not God—he is far away;
But someone that should be friend, lover, mother, priest, God all in one
And a stranger besides—who would not condemn nor interfere,
Who when everything is said from beginning to end
Would show the reason of it all
And tell you to go ahead
And work it out your own way. *

Have you ever wanted to help someone . . . a friend, family member, or neighbor? Have you ever experienced someone seeking your help, as is the 15-year-old girl in the poem? Have you ever tried to help someone who was having a personal, physical, emotional, or social problem? Let us assume that the following person requested your help.

Susan is a 20-year-old woman whom you know fairly well from your classes at the local university. Lately you notice that she has been withdrawn and preoccupied. One day after class she asks to talk with you. Finding a quiet place, Susan shares her feelings that her roommates dislike her. She thinks they are avoiding her, talking behind her back, and refusing to eat with her. She wants you to go back to the dorm with her and talk with them.

What are you to do? What would be the most helpful way for you to proceed in order to help Susan? What feelings do you have about helping her? What feelings do you have about her request for help? This chapter will enable you to learn about helping and your role as a helper in a social or professional realm.

HELPING—THE ART

Helping is one of the most common words in our vocabulary. As infants we were all totally dependent upon others. As we grew older, we became more capable of doing things for ourselves, and the way in which we depended upon others changed. Eventually we all experienced a partial role reversal and now are helpers ourselves as parents, friends, siblings, caretakers, breadwinners, etc. Certainly, how we fulfill these helping roles depends to an extent on our commitment and our desire to give of ourselves.

---

*From Hale, N. (1971). *Freud and the Americans: The beginnings of psychoanalysis.* New York: Oxford University Press, p. 412.

Helping—what is it? How is it defined? Some of us might say that help-ing is caring for another person or interceding in another person's life to make things easier for that person. There is no question that helping does infer these kinds of notions. But we also know that helping sometimes means letting go and not interceding. It literally means taking a "hands-off" approach and refraining from any involvement—physical or otherwise.

Wendy Miller is leaving the hospital today with her newborn son, Eric. Obviously, Eric is unable to care for himself, and it is Wendy's responsibility to do so. Wen-dy sees this as a welcome challenge and looks forward to helping Eric grow into a mature young man.

Helen Spence, a single parent, is the mother of a 20-year-old son in trouble for drug abuse. He also is unemployed and feels that his mother's responsibility is to help him with various problems as well as to pay all his expenses. Helen, however, has decided that Donald's behavior is unacceptable and that she can no longer assume responsibility for him. She tells him that she loves him very much and her decision to stop supporting him stems from that love. Helen informs Donald that he must leave her home and that she will no longer support him financially or bail him out of his brushes with the law over drug problems.

Helen and Wendy are both helping their children, but with different ap-proaches. There are a variety of ways to help people, and helping professionals must continue to remind themselves that each client's situation is unique and the approach to helping should address that uniqueness.

Simply defined, helping is a way of assisting someone who is in need (Cor-mier, Cormier, & Weisser, 1984). Helping by the very nature of the word in-volves relationship and interaction. "Relationship is an emotional experience" (Perlman, 1979, p. 5). Often, when our emotions are touched, we are moved to change. When we have a relationship with another person, it affirms our personhood—our worth as individuals. In helping relationships, whether they be social or professional, the message "I care about you" is being sent to the person being helped. Think for a moment about Jim Olin:

Jim is a 35-year-old journalist who has cared for and enjoyed his elderly father for the past 10 years. Jim's father has died very suddenly, and Jim's colleagues decide to actively help him work through the grieving process. They arrange to spend evenings with Jim, they send him cards, and most of all, they encourage Jim to talk about his father. Clearly, Jim is hearing the message, "We care about you," and he is able to share his feelings. The situation cannot be changed, but Jim feels better prepared to cope with his loss.

Helping also involves interaction. The person being helped feels the responsiveness of the helper. The person knows the helper cares and also knows the helper wants to help. Jim's colleagues clearly demonstrated their desire to help him—to respond to his need. Wendy certainly confirmed her response to her infant son. But what about Helen Spence—did she respond to her son's needs? It is important that helpers not confuse caring with being gentle and kind. Sometimes one must be firm and assertive. Even though we often say that people must learn to help themselves, this does not mean that this is done in isolation. People who interact with others and learn that others really care about them find that changing, though difficult, is not impossible.

HISTORICAL PERSPECTIVE

Helping throughout time has been influenced by certain people and key events. The art of helping is not new to this century. In fact, history is rich in examples of the nature of helping and how it affected the world. These early events of helping have influenced the way in which our society today responds to helping situations.

Since the beginning of time, people have been responsible for the care of children. In the first chapter of the Bible, we read about Cain and Abel and how they were cared for by Adam and Eve. From generation to generation our notions about growth and development and needs of children may change, but the major premise that children need caretakers remains constant. Hence, parenting may be the earliest form of helping.

There are particular individuals who have influenced the helping professions throughout the ages. An awareness of their contributions assists us as helpers to identify a true sense of our roots.

If we look at the first five chapters of the Old Testament of the Bible, we will find the fascinating story of how Moses, born about 1300 B.C., led his people from Egypt to Palestine—from slavery to freedom. We also will be reminded of the Ten Commandments, known as the "Torah of Moses." The Ten Commandments are laws that help us to lead our lives. Regardless of our religious beliefs, these laws still hold true today. They can assist us in our daily lives by showing us how to live with other people in a congenial and caring fashion. For many of us, these laws define certain rights and wrongs, such as: "Thou shalt not kill." They establish guidelines for each of us in our attempts to live productive, useful lives.

Hippocrates (460?–377? B.C.) formulated several important ideas concerning the practice of medicine. He believed that medical treatment should be dominated by logic and reason, not by superstition, which was prevalent during his life. Many of his ideas formulated the basis of Western medical practice during the 1800s. Perhaps his most famous contribution is the Hippocratic oath, still used by physicians today. In essence, this oath attests to the physician's responsibility to and sense of duty towards patients.

Socrates (469–399 B.C.) was one of the most important teachers throughout history. He believed that evil was a result of ignorance, not of some innate quality within the individual. Socrates devoted his life to finding the truth. He could be found teaching in the streets, the market place, and gymnasiums.

So influential was his teaching that he was condemned to death. Politicians feared his searches for truth.

Socrates taught people by using a questioning approach and encouraging people to think for themselves. This format is not unlike the educational process that occurs in informal helping. Helpers encourage clients to analyze situations, to seek out answers, and to find the truth. Socrates also has been credited as an early user of the inductive approach, in which he taught people to observe the particulars of a situation and eventually apply those observations to the entire situation. Inductive approaches, especially in research, continue to serve helping professionals as a valuable methodology for studying client problems.

Ancient Greece had famous events as well as people. We all remember that athletics, or the development of a sound body as well as mind, was an important concern to the Greeks. It is felt that the early Olympic Games were held to honor Greek gods and the death of heroes. These early games were considered sacred, and people from all parts of Greece participated despite political differences. Helpers of all disciplines recognize the importance of development of the body as well as the mind. We continue to strive to help the whole person.

In more modern times, helpers such as Florence Nightingale (1820–1910) also have served to influence particular professions. Nightingale is known as the founder of nursing. Born to a wealthy family, she was a well-educated woman who had to talk her parents into letting her study nursing.

Nightingale supervised a hospital and the nurses in that hospital during the Crimean War. She was acutely aware of sanitation problems, recognizing they were causing more deaths than the war. Her philosophy, which nursing continues to use today, posited that the prevention of illness is as important as the curing of disease. Nightingale returned to the United States at the end of the War and established better schools to prepare more qualified nurses.

Florence Nightingale has left a rich legacy to the profession of nursing. She was living proof that the art and science of nursing is critical to the wellbeing of patients. She used elementary research principles to collect data that later changed sanitation codes.

Nightingale's work continues to be the basis for much of today's practice. Her commitment to helping serves as a reminder to those who work in more comfortable and convenient health care settings—unlike the hospital in the Crimea.

Perhaps one of the most important psychologists and educators in modern times is Carl Rogers, who was born in 1903. Rogers's influence upon helping professions has been profound and widespread. He is best known for his work in client-centered therapy. He is credited with identifying the characteristics of a therapeutic environment—warmth, genuineness, concreteness, and empathy. Rogers believes that helpers must encourage clients to talk. He feels the counselor's or helper's role is purely to reflect the client's thoughts and feelings. Although many helpers might disagree, saying that more is expected of their role, most would agree that helping the client get "in touch" with feelings is essential to the helping relationship. Rogers has a worldwide reputation, and his beliefs about having clients express their feelings and creating environments conducive to helping are still highly respected.

The goals of helping have remained consistent throughout the ages. Helpers have continually demonstrated that the search for truth, frequently through knowledge, is essential for growth and independence.

THE GOALS OF HELPING

Carkhuff and Berenson (1977) identify four goals of helping:

- Client exploration
- Client understanding
- Client action
- Client learning.

Successfully encouraging a client to explore feelings is a major challenge to helping professionals. Many clients need to examine in depth feelings about particular problems or issues. This exploration can be painful, so much so that they may wish to terminate the relationship. Consider the case of Peter and his fiancee, Joyce:

> Peter is a 25-year-old engineer with an excellent job at a major company. He owns his own house and is quite settled in his life-style. Joyce, who is engaged to Peter, has lived with him for about a year. They have always talked of marriage, but Peter seems very hesitant about setting a date. Peter is attentive and loving towards Joyce; he does not see a need to be married. Joyce decides, however, that she needs more commitment and has told Peter that she is moving out of the state at the end of the month.
>
> Peter is devastated at this news; his life revolves around Joyce and their special relationship. He decides to talk to his minister, who knows both of them. The minister probes and encourages Peter to talk about marriage in general and what it means to him. Peter begins to answer and with further questioning talks about his parents' marriage. It is obvious that he is becoming quite upset as he recollects his childhood, his parents' bitter arguments, and how alone and frightened he felt. He is weeping as he recalls his father pointing a gun at him and his mother. Peter then goes on to explore his own behavior.

Exploration allows the client to move towards understanding. It helps to put the problems into perspective.

> Peter continues to see the minister on a weekly basis. He has realized that he is afraid of marriage because he would not want to subject his children to a similar childhood. Peter also continues to explore his own reactions to anger and admits

that he is more verbally abusive than physically abusive. He tends to retreat from arguments because he does not want to react like his father. He admits that retreating has often caused him trouble because he does not always confront problems.

Once the client has an understanding of the problems and what the choices are, a course of action can be pursued. Without question, getting the client to act—to do something about the problem—is an important goal of helping.

For Peter, seeking help from the minister is an impressive first step. It indicates that he wants to do something about his fears of marriage. He is not able, however, to resolve all of his conflict in a month's time, and Joyce moves away. Although this is painful for Peter, he continues to explore and eventually decides that he is not ready for marriage at this time.

The goal of helping is not to provide fairytale endings. It is to help clients cope with and adapt to life's dilemmas. Learning is a valuable outcome of the helping process. It prepares people for what is ahead. "The process of learning begins and ends with exploration, understanding, and action" (Carkhuff & Berenson, 1977, p. 155). It must be recognized that the four goals—exploration, understanding, action, and learning—are not discrete; they overlap and occur continuously throughout the process. Blocker (1966) further adds that the goals of helping are preventive in nature. Peter has learned a lot about his feelings and behaviors. As he talks to his minister on his final visit, he states that he looks forward to another close relationship and the possibility of marriage in the future. In his next relationship, he plans to be more honest about his past experiences, and he will never again become engaged unless he fully intends to marry (Fig. 5-1).

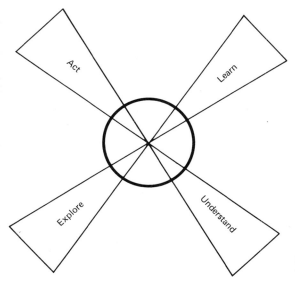

Figure 5-1. While professional helping involves four goals, it is frequently a blend of all.

SOCIAL HELPING RELATIONSHIPS

Throughout your lifetime you have observed and been involved in numerous helping relationships. Helping relationships in the universal and general sense are unwritten contracts and understandings between two or more people that involve interpersonal expressions of caring, concern, warmth, and emotional support. They assist the other person or group of people to grow emotionally, socially, spiritually, cognitively, and physically (Fig. 5–2). The persons being helped by the relationship may grow in all these aspects or just one. In other words, the person being helped finds the relationship growth-assisting, no matter how long or short its duration or how consistent or inconsistent its contact.

Your own family relationships may be a good example of a social helping process. Family members are frequently there to supervise your physical growth with the preparation of meals and to serve as emotional and social role models and support systems. Other significant human helping contacts are friends and elders who help you to continue this life growth process by introducing you to numerous life situations (Fig. 5–3). Through school you meet peers your own age and develop friendships that may continue through a lifetime.

You may recall the first example in this chapter, the example of Susan and your social relationship with her. You have gotten to know Susan rather

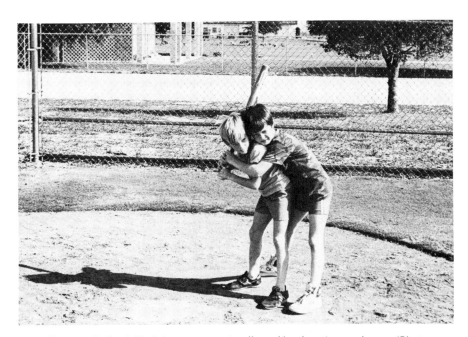

Figure 5-2. Social helping comes naturally and begins at an early age. *(Photo credit to Win Hames.)*

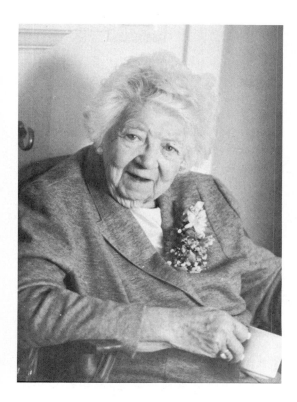

Figure 5-3. For many, the rewards of helping continue into the "golden" years. *(Photo credit to Peggy Haggerty.)*

spontaneously through your classes together. You know each other well enough to find it helpful to study together. Yours is a relationship in which you provide each other with emotional support and teach each other about the course content. Up until Susan's recent problem, you have mutually and equally shared your concerns about college courses and social life. You know Susan well enough to notice when she acts differently, and you care enough about her to take the time to listen to her problem. You are not a professional, and your relationship with her serves a rather spontaneous purpose of mutual companionship. You and Susan have never discussed when your relationship will end or how frequently you will see each other. All this has happened quite naturally.

Consider a grandfather teaching his grandson how to carve a wooden whistle. The grandfather's and grandson's relationship has developed due to normal family ties and mutual admiration and respect for each other. The grandfather is proud of his grandson's youth and intelligence. He hopes and believes that his grandson will carry on and replenish the family's good name and standing in the community. The grandson reciprocates this fondness and has a similar interest in working with his hands and working with wood. While the grandfather teaches the grandson how to carve a whistle, they enjoy the

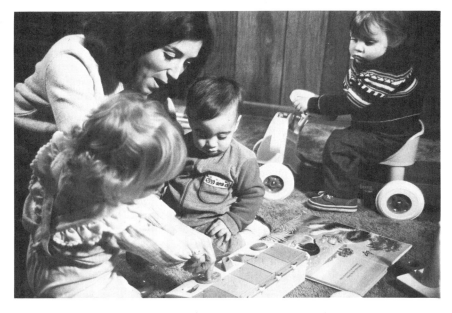

Figure 5-4. Helping—in a professional or a social setting—is a commitment to caring. *(Photo credit to Steve DeRosa.)*

emotional warmth of companionship and the satisfaction of successfully making something together. They mutually and equally respond to each other. Each hopes to continue the relationship ad infinitum.

Thus, the human process of a helping relationship is available in our society in numerous forms and in any number of situations and settings. Relationships vary in duration and frequency of time, degree of spontaneity, and purpose. The social helping relationship seems to be the foundation upon which our cultures are based so that the human race can be protected, improved, and reproduced (Fig. 5–4). It is underlying the theme in such songs as "No Man Is An Island," "I'll Never Walk Alone," "You Light Up My Life," and "Reach Out and Touch Somebody." Perhaps you can think of some personal life experiences in which this type of helping relationship has occurred.

PROFESSIONAL HELPING RELATIONSHIPS

Helping relationships in the professional context occur between a client and professional and contain many of the qualities of a social relationship. Social and professional relationships have in common the components of care, concern, development of trust, and attainment of growth or some other change in behavior, attitude, or feeling. The professional helping relationship is the foundation and core upon which professionals, especially in the health areas, fulfill their goals of assisting the individual, family, and community to change behavior in an attempt to attain the highest possible level of adaptation.

There are some major differences in the social and professional helping relationships. In contrast to social helping, the professional's services are specific in purpose, focused on the client, not based on friendship, unequal in interpersonal exchange, usually for a fee, and designed to be time-limited. Let us further discuss these differences (Table 5-1).

Professional versus Social Helping

The professional helping relationship does not usually occur spontaneously, as do many social relationships. The professional relationship develops with a specific purpose and goal, and with the client in mind. The professional helper responds to the client with attention and concern in hopes of developing trust and a working relationship. The professional intervenes, using therapeutic communication skills in a supportive, honest, and understanding manner so that the client is the major person who expresses him- or herself and is the major person who is helped. The professional works with the client to set up the goals, conditions, and limitations of the relationship. Therefore, unlike social relationships, the professional helping relationship places unequal focus on the helper and client.

Another difference in the social and professional relationship is the unequal amount of personal exchange between client and helper in the latter relationship. The client reveals personal information, while the helper listens and reveals information pertaining to the professional role and the services that can be provided. In a social relationship the persons may equally reveal information about themselves, and each member is being helped by the rela-

TABLE 5-1. COMPARISONS OF SOCIAL AND PROFESSIONAL RELATIONSHIPS

	Social	Professional
Self-disclosure	Mutual	Client disclosure
Communication	Chitchat	Therapeutic
Focus	Undirected, impersonal	Directed, personal
Cost	Free	Fee (usually)
Time	Unlimited— past, present, future	Limited— present
Goals	Unidentified; friendship, enjoyment	Identified; client learning, exploring, understanding, acting
Environment	Casual, spontaneous	Structured, planned

tionship. This is not to say that professionals do not receive satisfaction or benefits from their helping relationships. For many, a profession is a way of satisfying oneself emotionally and intellectually.

The professional can earn a living from fees collected from such relationships. However, not all professionals require a fee for service. Of course, in a social relationship the persons do not pay a monetary fee. The only payment is the time and energy that one puts into the relationship and the satisfaction one gains from it. Thus, the professional's satisfaction is secondary in nature.

Another major difference is that although the professional relationship contains the components of caring and concern, it is not built upon friendship but rather upon the client's needs. The professional helping relationship is one in which the client's real needs are uncovered. Unlike that of the social helping relationship, the focus of interactions is not on friendship. This does not preclude the helper from being friendly towards the client. Friendship, however, is not the goal of the professional helping relationship. The helper must strive to maintain an objective attitude in which the client's attitudes and feelings can be appreciated.

Much has been discussed and written about the extent to which one "gets involved" with clients. There are not many firm guidelines for specific behaviors that the helper accepts as professionally appropriate behavior. Some general guidelines can be found in the professional standards and ethical codes. Certainly, professionals bring their unique personalities to the professional arena. Some professionals are more friendly than others toward their clients. Others are more direct in their therapeutic responses and recommendations. As long as the professional helper objectively helps the client to attain independence in a responsible fashion, the helper's actions are considered appropriate.

A professional relationship not only emphasizes objectivity in helping the client, but the focus is such that the client is helped to increase independence. The client is taught to solve problems by defining the problem, assessing information, and setting goals, as well as deciding how to intervene and make the best use of available resources. In many social relationships, independence of function is not always the focus, and involved persons may become dependent upon each other in either a healthy or unhealthy fashion. It is important for the professional to prevent unhealthy dependence, whereas in the social relationship the degree of dependency is decided upon by the participants.

In a professional relationship, the client's ultimate responsibility is to change. Keep in mind the familiar saying, "You can lead a horse to water, but you cannot make it drink." The professional helper cannot make the client change. Professional helping relationships are successful only to the point that both parties are willing to work for change. It is important, in defining the scope of such a relationship, to establish mutually the needs and objectives to be met and to agree upon interventions. To facilitate this process, frequent evaluation of progress or lack of progress is constructive.

The professional helper realizes that others—for example, the family and community—are capable of helping, and in many cases better suited to help, the client. Professional helpers need to learn referral techniques and be familiar with community resources. A professional helper cannot expect to be "all things to all people." One must be cognizant of one's capabilities and limitations.

Professional helping relationships always have time constraints. Both parties should agree on the starting and finishing times of each session. At the conclusion, the relationship is evaluated, and termination is discussed. Often in social relationships the beginning and ending of relationships are uncertain and open-ended. People often say, "I'll see you later," with no strong commitment to follow through. By not being specific about a time or date as to when they will see you, they have not made a commitment. Thus, persons involved in a social relationship are not always totally honest about their commitments or responsibilities. In summary, the social relationship is less structured than the professional one, with no definite time, place, duration, or limit on the contacts, while the professional helping relationship is a purposefully directed activity involving interpersonal exchange between a helper and a client.

Influence of Helpers on Clients

Helpers do exert a certain amount of power over the attitudes and actions of clients. This power is not coercive in nature. Helpers do not try to punish or threaten clients in attempts to make them change their behavior (Janis, 1983). Professional helpers often do attempt to influence client behavior in an effort to help the clients improve. It is not unusual for the physician and the physical therapist to explain the type of therapy and the potential benefits to a client. This influence may be strong enough to induce the client to follow through with a therapeutic regime. Tedeschi and Lindskold (1976) report that influence is more effective than coercion when attempting to help people.

Summary

In conclusion, the focus of the professional helping relationship is on the client's needs in the biophysical, psychosocial, and/or cognitive modes. In this relationship, the helper assists the client through the problem-solving process in assessing needs and planning for effective intervention. Action is initiated by the client, the professional, or other significant members of the family and helping team. The ultimate goal is to assist the client in attaining and maintaining the highest possible level of health and independence.

STAGES IN PROFESSIONAL HELPING

Helping relationships mature through several stages of development. To facilitate the growth of helping relationships, professionals should have an understanding of these stages and be able to anticipate the feelings and behaviors

STAGE I: TRUST FORMATION

Trust is built upon consistency, positive regard, honesty, respect and empathy

STAGE II: RESISTANCE

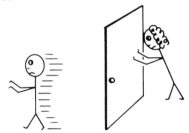

Client pulls back, helper shows concern

STAGE III: WORKING

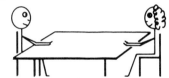

Client and helper are actively involved

STAGE IV: TERMINATION

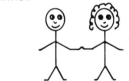

Figure 5-5. Stages in professional helping.

Saying goodbye – handshake – and good wishes

that are common. These stages are: trust formation, resistance, working phase, and termination (Fig. 5–5).

Trust Formation

The pivotal element in any meaningful relationship is trust. Rogers (1951) defines trust as consistency of words and actions. "There is no such thing as an automatic right to be trusted; it is a privilege that one earns" (Curtin, 1982, p. 98). Therefore, one of the purposes of the initial encounter is to begin fostering the development of trust. This is conveyed by verbal and nonverbal messages that are consistent with each other.

Sharon is a high school student who is talking to her guidance counselor, Mrs. Simpson, about her parents' marital problem. She knows that her mother would be upset if she told anyone about the home situation. Her father's alcohol problem is a great source of embarrassment, and she is expected to act as though this problem does not exist. She decides to talk to Mrs. Simpson about her home life because she feels counselors are appropriate people to talk to.

When Sharon enters the office, Mrs. Simpson invites her to sit down and share her thoughts. At first Sharon thinks Mrs. Simpson is interested, but then she notices that Mrs. Simpson keeps glancing at her watch and looking very inattentive. Sharon quickly picks up on the counselor's nonverbal behavior and decides not to tell her the real problems. Although Mrs. Simpson stated her interest in Sharon, her behavior indicated otherwise.

The client's trust is contingent upon the congruency of our communication and behavior (Parsons & Sandford, 1979). We must mean what we say and do as we say for a sense of security to develop. The client then feels safe from being ridiculed or judged and can begin to discuss topics that are other than superficial.

How do you create a trusting environment? There is no one specific answer to this question. Since all clients are unique, the method used varies from individual to individual. There are, however, certain common elements that enhance the development of a trusting relationship. They are as follows:

1. *The helper's approach must be consistent.* The client must be able to feel the helper's "presence" and sense that the helper is truly interested. The client needs to know that within established, realistic parameters, the helper will be there when needed. Look for a moment at the very first trusting rapport developed in life.

Jeffrey, age 3 months, has established a strong bond with his mother and knows that when he cries she will pick him up, feed him, or change his diaper. He is secure in his mother's care.

Helping involves meeting both physical and psychological needs. In this example, the mother may hold the baby close to her body, sing a lullaby, or rock the baby, thereby meeting his psychological, as well as physical needs.

In a professional relationship the client must have a sense that the helper can be depended upon. The client must know that the helper is available and concerned about what happens.

2. *The helper must have a positive regard for the client.* The term "positive regard" means respect for the client without judging the client's actions. If a helper feels superior to a client, there is a tendency to assume an authoritarian role. A helper who takes this approach is not enhancing trust development. The helper who respects the client for being a worthwhile human being is more apt to encourage a trusting relationship.

It is important to note here that not passing judgment upon a client's value system does not mean that you, personally, agree with everything the client says or does. Rather, it means that you will refrain from employing your value system when helping the client. "Positive regard in interpersonal processes is defined . . . as a respect and concern for the helpee's feelings, experiences and potentials" (Carkhuff & Berenson, 1977, p. 11). Consider the following:

> Adam Nichols is explaining to his science teacher why he cheated on the last exam. Adam is truly sorry about what has happened and decides that he must confess his actions to his teacher. Although his teacher, Mr. Jones, does not condone cheating, he listens to Adam and praises him for coming forward and being honest.

3. *The helper must always be honest with the client.* The trust developed in a helping relationship is mutual. The client, as well as the helper, is responsible for responding in an open, honest manner. Often the helper is confused or baffled by what the client says. To pretend that you understand the client's message, when in essence you have no idea about what is being said, takes away from the sincerity of the process. Clients seek helpers because they have a need, and if the helper begins to comment about the client's problems without really understanding them, the client quickly recognizes the dishonesty.

Sometimes honesty demands a steadfast and serious approach, and at other times it calls for a more humorous one (Fig. 5–6). Humor helps us to see incongruities; it helps us to identify the absurd. "Humor does not necessarily mean joking or teasing. . . . the put-down of another" (Murray, 1983, p. 192).

> Leanna confides to her lifelong friend Gail that things in her marriage are not going well. During a Saturday night get-together with several couples, Leanna and her husband have an argument in front of everyone. Her husband storms out of the house in a rage. Gail assumes a supportive position, staying with Leanna as the rest of the couples leave. Several people mumble quick goodbyes and hasten to leave. One guest claims he has had a lovely evening.
>
> After they all leave, Gail listens to a weeping Leanna. She appears devastated as she talks about her friends and how awful the evening must have been for them. Gail quietly reminds her, "Well, one man had a 'lovely' time." The two of them—Gail and Leanna—roar with laughter. It feels good.

"You lose when you cannot expand your mind with humor. You dry up emotionally, and you have lost an opportunity to learn, to mature, and to enjoy" (Murray, 1983, p. 192).

4. *The helper must respect the confidentiality of the client.* A trust relationship occurs once the client has taken the risk to share something that is very meaningful and personal. The client rightly assumes that such information is confidential. If you feel that you have a moral or ethical obligation to share something the client has told you, be honest and explain why you must do so. Have you ever asked a friend not to tell something to anyone and 2 weeks later found out that everyone knows? If you have, you can appreciate how terrible a client feels when a helper cannot be trusted.

5. *The helper must have an empathetic understanding of the client.* "Em-

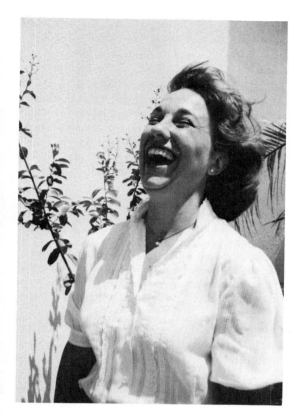

Figure 5-6. Humor is often a tension releaser and most therapeutic. *(Photo credit to Peggy Haggerty.)*

pathy is an attempt to perceive the world as the client does" (Fritz, Russell, Wilcox, & Shirk, 1984, p. 51). It occurs when the helper tries to put him- or herself in the "shoes" of the client in an attempt to develop an appreciation of the client's world and feelings. Egan (1982) suggests that an empathetic approach enables helpers to establish a relationship in which clients will effectively work on problem solving.

"Empathy is both an attitude and a skill" (Cormier, Cormier, & Weisser, 1984, p. 22). An empathetic attitude reflects the helper's desire to understand the client's world from the clients frame of reference. As helpers develop expertise, they are able to communicate this attitude to clients. Once this is communicated, the client senses that the helper is interested and understands what is happening.

Empathy is not to be confused with sympathy. Sympathy is feeling sorry for the client. Helpers throughout the years have been told that sympathy is never appropriate. The implication has been that it is too emotionally charged and leads to involvement beyond the parameters of a helping profession. One's tendency may indeed be to do something for the person rather than to encourage him or her to take action. Sympathy, felt too frequently and too deeply, can be emotionally draining and energy-depleting, but it is a very human feeling and most legitimate. It need not be denied, simply channeled. Consider the following:

> Allysin Yates is a physical therapist who has been working diligently with Mr. Harper, a 55-year-old victim of a stroke. In the past 3 months she has watched Mr. Harper progress to the point where he is ready to go back to work. Allysin is quite happy for Mr. Harper because she knows that his wife and two teenage children have really suffered during this crisis. Since Mr. Harper is the bread-winner, their financial resources have been depleted. Yet neither the family nor Mr. Harper complained; they were happy they had one another and that Mr. Harper was alive.
>
> Mr. Harper comes for his regular 3 o'clock session and is quite upset. His employer has told him that his job has been dissolved and there is no available position to give him. Mr. Harper is distraught; he keeps saying, "My poor family—what will they do for money?"
>
> Although Allysin feels empathetic, she also is sympathetic. Mr. Harper and his family have worked so hard; it does not seem fair. Allysin is able to attend to Mr. Harper's concerns in a professional manner, but she knows that this is one patient whom she will never forget. She realizes how sorry she feels for this patient.

To summarize, trust is a fundamental element in all helping relationships. Do not assume that a client will trust you because you are in the role of helper. Trust is reciprocal; both the client and the helper must earn the trust of the other.

Helping relationships are built upon the consistency of our day-to-day encounters with clients. Clients will only begin to discuss their deepest and most meaningful thoughts and feelings after they are certain that the helper can be trusted! (Fig. 5–7)

This discussion of trust might seem elementary to you, since you may feel that all clients have the right to expect a trustful rapport with a helper. However, in 1972 the American Hospital Association presented to the general public the Patient's Bill of Rights. This statement was presented to assure the consumer of health, better hospital care, and more satisfaction with this care.

This bill has implications for all helping professionals, not only those working in hospital settings. In essence, this document describes the inalienable rights to privacy, confidentiality, and knowledge. For a complete description of the Patient's Bill of Rights, see Appendix III.

Resistance

Initial ambivalence or trepidation about sharing significant feelings is to be expected in a new relationship. This uncertainty is indicative of the resistance stage. The client has made an initial investment in the helping relationship, but may be hesitant to continue or is unsure of how much commitment to make. Sometimes one must commit a great deal of time and undergo finan-

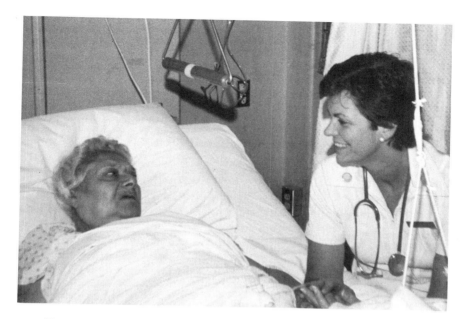

Figure 5-7. Eye contact, touch, and good listening skills are simple but valuable ways of gaining trust. *(Photo credit to Dayle Joseph.)*

cial loss, physical and emotional pain, and embarrassment in order to increase his or her adaptation. It is only natural to consider how much one is willing and able to give for that end.

Many avoidance-type behaviors are indicative of resistance. Changing the subject, questioning the competency of the professional, discussing superficial social issues, being late or absent, or appearing uninterested are all to be expected. By being understanding, supportive, and trustworthy, the helper can encourage the client to increase involvement and to move into the working stage of the relationship.

Working

The third stage is the major part of the helping relationship and is a crucial factor in increasing the client's adaptation. The helper and the client are both committed to actively plan and implement solutions to the identified problems during this stage.

Those clients who are actively working to resolve problems seem to have increased physical and emotional involvement. As they begin to reveal themselves and their vulnerabilities, they may experience a heightened anxiety, but this is manageable as long as trust exists. Frequently the relationship becomes more collaborative and the client can be more objective. She or he is relaxed and self-confident enough to look beyond her- or himself. Increased independence is a result of professional helping and a goal of this stage.

Professionals are most helpful during this time if they continue to respond in an honest, empathetic way, using therapeutic communication skills. Comfortable disagreement is healthy as the client explores possibilities and understands unsuccessful actions. It is part of the professional's role to comment on the client's changes in behavior, reinforce the client's strengths, point out overall progress, and encourage independent participation in self-improvement.

Termination of Relationships

Helpers spend a lot of time learning how to establish and maintain professional relationships. They also need to learn how to end relationships—to terminate in the right manner at the right time. Ideally, termination heralds a positive aspect for the client, indicating he or she has reached a higher level of adaptation and can now cope independently. But sometimes this is not the case. Sometimes the client's adaptation has diminished and care is being transferred to another helper.

Saying goodbye is difficult for both the helper and the client. A special rapport has often developed. Both might be wondering how the client will manage, but if it has been determined that the client is ready, or otherwise needs to leave, then it is important for the helper to support and encourage that decision. It is hoped the time of termination is known and can be planned for, as in the case of a hospitalized patient who is admitted for a given number of days. At other times, termination may be in the distant, unknown future, or it may occur suddenly and unexpectedly. It is helpful, therefore, to discuss termination briefly in the first meeting and in more detail during subsequent meetings.

Many of us treat goodbyes with special reverence because we know we cannot ever again create the same situation. Sometimes the helper merely says a friendly farewell wishing the client the best. At other times a deep attachment has occurred and the helper may decide something special is in order.

> Alice Farmer, a college professor, has just completed a year teaching five honors students philosophy. It has been an exciting year for both Alice and her students. She decides to write each of them an individualized poem to remind them of this eventful year.
>
> Mary Foster is a surgical nurse who has cared for Mrs. Smith, a 75-year-old amputee, for 2 months. Mary has cared for her almost daily and is very fond of her. When Mrs. Smith is discharged, Mary shakes her hand and lightly kisses her on the forehead. Mrs. Smith is touched—she knows this has been a special relationship.

Occasionally the reverse situation occurs and the client feels the relationship has been especially meaningful. In this case, "The client may give a gift . . . in an effort to convey feelings of appreciation, warmth, caring, and to leave an object that ensures being remembered" (Murray, 1983, p. 207). It is not unusual for professionals to feel awkward about accepting gifts. Helpers know that many clients cannot afford gifts and do not expect anything more than their salaries. It may be wise to accept the gift, however. Refusal can be interpreted as a rejection of the client.

> Sally Tyler, a nutritionist who does diet counseling, is seeing Rachael Gillis for her last session on weight loss. Rachel has lost 50 pounds in 6 months' time and is feeling terrific about her will power and her new appearance. She recognizes Sally's ability and knows that she has done so well because Sally has listened to all of her problems. Rachael has learned several new, easy recipes over the past 6 months. She decides to compile them in a book for Sally. Rachael tells Sally that she wants her to share these recipes with other clients. Sally enthusiastically accepts the gift and later writes Rachael a short note explaining how often she has used the recipes.

As the time for termination nears, helpers must assume the responsibility for preparing patients—"talk about feelings—yours and the other person's—as well as about realistic discharge and teaching plans" (Murray, 1983, p. 207). Begin to evaluate by pointing out ways in which the patient has grown. Be realistic about the client's response. Some clients will be happy because they will feel "well" and capable again—ready to face the world. Others may be sad or angry because they know the work has not been accomplished and time has run out.

> Fern Thornton is a 45-year-old patient assigned to a chronic hospital ward. In the past 3 months, Fern has enjoyed a warm relationship with a young student psychotherapist. In fact, Fern is actually talking to this student; prior to this time she had not talked in 5 years. About a month before leaving, the student approaches the topic of terminating. From that day on Fern refuses to talk.

The student feels disappointed; however, the patient obviously is even more distressed. Even though we are not happy with the consequences of being honest and discussing termination, we have a moral obligation to do so.

THE CLIENT'S FEELINGS

People who ask for help generally are having some kind of trouble—marital, job, illness, or other. For some, needing professional help may be a new experience. For most, it is a threatening one. Astute helpers can anticipate some common feelings and behaviors in clients.

First of all, "people who have a problem feel it uniquely" (Perlman, 1979, p. 52). Each may think he or she is the only person who has ever grieved so deeply, hurt so badly, been treated so unjustly. Some may be very skeptical about seeking assistance for just that reason—"no one could possibly under-stand." Interestingly, most people are not looking for someone to solve their problems. They simply want someone to listen, care, and understand. They earnestly want someone to talk to who is not going to pass judgment on them or think less of them because of their plight.

Revealing inner thoughts and feelings can be a painful process. Very often, if not always, this process involves disclosing significant information—perhaps, information unknown to the rest of the world (Adler & Towne, 1981). For many, self-disclosure is an invasion of privacy, with the resultant risk that the listener will reject them because of their feelings or behavior. Some people may feel guilty, especially those who were brought up to believe they were never to tell certain things to anyone. For some, asking for help may be more embarrassing than risky. Those patients with health problems often avoid seek-ing help because they are embarrassed or feel foolish discussing distressing symptoms that relate to certain bodily functions. Furthermore, clients may interpret this sharing of feelings as a weakness. It may represent their inability to solve their own problems. For many cultural groups, this may represent failure.

Sometimes clients, even those who desperately want help, may hesitate. They feel uncomfortable, fearing they might learn something they do not want to know. Patients who seek help from physicians often put off this need until the physical problem becomes overwhelming. These patients often fear they have a dread disease or will suffer pain if the disease is treated. Other clients are somewhat insecure about asking for help. These are the people who give indirect cues and hope that the astute helper will ask them what is the matter.

Consequently, many people resist professional help. They do not like revealing their concerns and feeling exposed or dependent. Some may even be openly angry and hostile. Some continually avoid discussing the real issue. Others are just unable to reveal their thoughts. These clients are the helper's real challenges! Perhaps we can be more effective by better understanding the art of asking for help. By recognizing how difficult this is, we may be more empathetic and encouraging to those who shy from our assistance.

A few clients feel professional help will provide magical cures for prob-lems. These clients have unrealistic expectations and often do not recognize that they must assume responsibility for solving their own problems. They send messages to the helper such as "Help me, mother me, take care of me, cure me." These clients have a need to be dependent upon the helper. Some may continually ask for more help or refuse to participate in necessary self-treat-ment and care. It is important for the helper to promote independence as con-structively as possible. Helpers need to enhance security and supportively praise success in an effort to increase the client's level of adaptation.

Not all clients, however, react negatively to helping. Many feel that help-ing encounters are what enables them to continue to cope with problems. They feel these relationships are supportive and often comment on the pleasure and success the relationship has brought them. Clients feel that they can self-disclose and share their innermost secrets. They understand the helper's role and recognize that a therapeutic relationship is not risky—that helpers do not judge their behavior. Clients feel a potential for growth. In essence, many clients appreciate the need to purge their souls and know that they can begin again.

Thus, clients have various feelings about asking for and receiving professional help. But if their needs and feelings are accepted in a nonjudgmental way by an empathetic helper, most do experience a sense of relief that help is attainable.

THE HELPER'S FEELINGS

The most successful helpers are those who are in touch with their feelings. People who are new at helping are often confused about what to do with their feelings and their reactions to clients. They may feel their role is to be detached and distant—always in control. It quickly becomes apparent that being an effective professional helper necessitates involvement with people. To deny feelings would be dishonest and not in the best interests of the client. Helpers are human and have likes and dislikes, joys and sorrows. It is appropriate to have these feelings and even to express them. It is inappropriate to allow these feelings to interfere with a client's progress, however.

One of the most important lessons for young professional helpers to learn is to "be you—be real." If you are confused, admit it. If you are sad, cry. If you are excited, share that. But always do what you do with discretion and honestly.

The mother of a young child who has just died of a malignant brain tumor sees one of her son's nurses attempting to conceal her crying. The mother's response is to hug the nurse and say, "We always knew you cared for Jeff, but seeing you cry leaves us with no doubt. It helps."

In some situations, countertransference may occur and interfere with helping. This involves the unconscious desire on the part of the helper not to assist the client for personal reasons. This response is specific for an individual helper and is inappropriate in the helping relationship. Sometimes "feelings are 'transferred' from the helper's own past relationships with significant people to the present helper relationship" (Brammer, 1979, p. 29). As long as the helper realizes these feelings and responds appropriately, the client can still be helped. If the client reminds the helper of another person, extra effort may be needed not to confuse this present relationship with a past one or a different one. If the helper finds the client's personality distasteful, heightened objectivity may help. We do not have to like people to care for them. However, we do have to respect their right to receive care. In extreme situations it may be best to find another helper for the client.

Another potentially harmful situation occurs when a helper allows his or her sense of power and authority to dominate. It is only natural for a successful helper to feel good about the progress of clients. There is a certain amount of pride associated with a job well done. These feelings are very normal and all helpers have them—even though admitting to having them may be difficult. But because many clients are dependent at some point upon the helper, there is the risk that this may be fostered to meet the ego needs of the helper, not the needs of the client. Conscientious helpers strive to keep these feelings in check as they recognize that clients benefit most from egalitarian relationships.

Consider the master teacher who is observing the student teacher. Clearly, the job of the master teacher is to be critical and to point out areas that need improvement. However, the master teacher who uses this role to exert undue influence and power over the student is not, in fact, being helpful or supportive of the student's learning experience.

Professional helping can be an exhausting responsibility. Helpers are not always physically or emotionally prepared to help one hundred percent of the time.

> Think for a moment about Harry Knowlton, a physical therapist. Harry has spent the weekend skiing, having lots of fun enjoying the social life as well as the slopes. Now it is 8:30 Monday morning, and Harry is less than enthusiastic about doing routine exercises with Mr. Blais, a paraplegic. Harry, however, is sensitive to Mr. Blais's needs as well as being aware of his own feelings. Harry works extra hard that morning because he knows he has a professional obligation, although he willingly admits, "I'd rather be skiing."

We all have moments when we do not feel like helping—this is normal. We need to recognize these feelings and, in cases when they are overwhelming, to postpone helping. Handling our own personal stresses can deplete our energy for helping others (Murray, 1983).

We also need to be responsible about helping ourselves and caring for our own needs. Burnout, the process by which our professional energy is permanently depleted, can easily occur. All helpers require time away from helping situations to tend to their own needs.

> Ralph Epstien has been a counselor for several years in a large high school. When he leaves the school at 5 P.M., Ralph makes a conscious effort not to bring the students' problems home with him. He spends his evenings with his family working on household projects, playing games with his children, or reading a book. Ralph's students know that he is available between 9 A.M. and 4:30 P.M. His door is always open. His private life, however, belongs to him, and students are not encouraged to call or contact Ralph during his "free" hours.

Burnout may be avoided by not overextending oneself. Maintaining healthy dietary and sleep patterns as well as work hours are essential. An occasional late night at work is to be expected, but allowing this to happen too frequently is self-destructive. Responsible professionals need keen cognitive skills, sharp observations, and physical stamina. They should be emotionally stable, and this requires social and emotional outlets. It is helpful to share professional conflicts and problems with colleagues. At other times, socialization becomes a priority and "shop talk" is inappropriate.

ETHICAL CONSIDERATIONS

It would be inappropriate to end a discussion of professional helping without some attention being given to ethical decision making. As human beings we all have feelings, beliefs, and values, and they influence the way we practice our professions. When in doubt, our natural tendency is to do what we personally believe is best or to choose what we think is most important. Sometimes it is not clear what is best for our client. When decisions must be made under these circumstances, our most difficult challenge is not to impose our own value system on others. Ethical decision making should be a shared process based upon mutual respect. Knowing and understanding the client's beliefs and values becomes critical. Ethical dilemmas involve situations where one must choose between two or more equally satisfactory or unsatisfactory alternatives. Choosing the alternative that is most consistent with the client's values or supporting the client to do the same is sometimes quite difficult, but it is paramount for professional pride, responsibility, and accountability.

Professionals also have moral obligations to clients. Clients rightfully deserve the best care possible, and as helping professionals we have a commitment to give that care. Many professions establish codes or guidelines (see Appendix IV for one example, the American Nurses' Association Code of Ethics). These serve as creeds representing the highest ideals of care, and remind helpers that clients are "vulnerable and must depend upon the professional's special knowledge and skills" (Benjamin & Curtis, 1981, p. 6).

Codes also help to remind us that our conduct must be beyond reproach. Professionals have access to very personal information, and they must ensure that the client's privacy is always maintained. We also must continually maintain our skills and update our knowledge base. Clients deserve helpers who can offer the latest in scientific techniques and approaches. Moreover, they deserve helpers who are competent and safe practitioners.

Paul Miller, the local pharmacist, notes that Alex Loiselle has three different pain prescriptions from three different doctors. Alex is an elderly man who often seems mildly confused. Paul knows that he has been treated at a local clinic and feels that the doctors may not have been aware of one another's prescriptions. Although each prescription could legally be filled, Paul calls the three physicians involved and gets an order for one pain medication.

Paul has acted responsibly and ethically, demonstrating a concern for Mr. Loiselle. Paul knows that he is accountable for his actions and feels that his refusal to fill three prescriptions was in the patient's best interest.

"Codes of ethics . . . have existed since Hippocrates, but they are no more than professional suggestions to colleagues about how to behave" (Frommer, 1981, p. 309). Each of you, as beginning helpers, should become familiar with the creed of your profession and establish your own moral guidelines for client care.

IMPORTANT REMINDERS

1. Helping relationships in both social and professional contexts share common characteristics of interpersonal caring, concern, and warmth. There are distinct differences, however, between the two types of relationships that need to be understood by professional helpers. Both social and professional relationships are growth producing.
2. Professional helping is client oriented for the purpose of fostering independence and enhancing adaptation. Clients are assisted to explore and understand their situations, learn new coping strategies, and act upon problem-solving decisions.
3. There are four stages of a helping relationship—trust formation, resistance, working phase, and termination. The helper intervenes in a manner that effectively assists the client through these stages.
4. Each client brings unique feelings and needs to a relationship. Professional helpers can facilitate problem management by fully assessing and incorporating these uniquenesses.
5. Each professional has unique feelings, characteristics, and needs. These must be recognized and addressed appropriately if one is to be an effective, objective professional helper.
6. Vital to all professional helping relationships are trust and ethical conduct.

REFERENCES

Adler, R. B., & Towne, N. (1981). *Looking out/looking in* (3rd ed.). New York: Holt, Rinehart & Winston.

Benjamin, M., & Curtis, J. (1981). *Ethics in nursing.* New York: Oxford University Press.

Blocker, D. H. (1966). *Developmental counseling.* New York: Ronald Press.

Brammer, L. M. (1979). *The helping relationship process and skills.* Englewood Cliffs, N.J.: Prentice-Hall.

Carkhuff, R. R., & Berenson, B. G. (1977). *Beyond counseling and therapy* (2nd ed.). New York: Holt, Rinehart & Winston.

Cormier, L. S., Cormier, W. H., & Weisser, R. J. (1984). *Interviewing and helping skills for health professionals.* Monterey, Calif.: Wadsworth Health Sciences Division.

Curtin, L. (1982). The commitment of nursing. In L. Curtin & M. J. Flaherty (Eds.), *Nursing ethics—theories and pragmatics.* Bowie, Md.: Robert J. Brady.

Egan, G. (1982). *The skilled helper* (2nd ed.). Monterey, Calif.: Brooks/Cole.

Fritz, P., Russell, C., Wilcox, E., & Shirk, F. (1984). *Interpersonal communication in nursing: An interactionist approach.* E. Norwalk, Conn.: Appleton-Century-Crofts.

Frommer, M. J. (1981). *Ethical issues in health care.* St. Louis: C. V. Mosby.

Hale, N. (1971). *Freud and the Americans: The beginning of psychoanalysis.* New York: Oxford University Press. Poem of a 15-year-old girl originally printed in 1916 in Margaret Anderson's avant-garde *The Little Review.*

Janis, I. L. (1983). *Short-term counseling guidelines based on recent research.* New Haven: Yale University Press.

Murray, R. B. (1983). The helping relationship. In R. B. Murray & M. M. W. Huelskoetter (Eds.), *Psychiatric mental health nursing giving emotional care.* Englewood Cliffs, N. J.: Prentice-Hall.

Parsons, V., & Sandford, N. (1979). *Interpersonal interaction in nursing.* Menlo Park, N.J.: Addison-Wesley.

Perlman, H. H. (1979). *Relationship.* Chicago: University of Chicago Press.

Rogers, C. (1951). The interpersonal relationship: The core of guidance. In J. Stewart (Ed.), *Bridges, not walls* (2nd ed.). Reading, Mass.: Addison-Wesley.

Tedeschi, J. T., & Lindskold, S. (1976). *Social psychology: Interdependence, interaction, and influence.* New York: Wiley.

People don't get along because they fear each other.
People fear each other because they don't know each other.
They don't know each other because they have not properly communicated
with each other.

                                        Martin Luther King, Jr.

6

Communication

Upon completion of the following reading and suggested exercises, the student will be able to:
1. Define the term *communication.*
2. Discuss the theoretical components of the communication process.
3. Define direct and indirect feedback.
4. Describe distractors that interfere with the communication process.
5. Identify where distractors can occur in the communication process.
6. Compare and contrast verbal and nonverbal communication.
7. Describe the usefulness of touch, sight, sound, and smell in assessing nonverbal behavior.
8. Identify the basic principles of written communication.

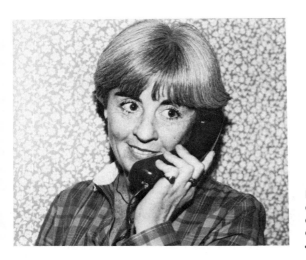

Figure 6-1. Communication occurs in many forms. What kind of a message is this woman receiving? (*Photo credit to Ron Joseph.*)

COMMUNICATION—THE PROCESS

Communication is the basis for our existence. If our ability to communicate were lost, our lives would become barren. Can you imagine what it would be like to live in a society in which there is no exchange of thoughts, feelings, words, or ideas? Can you imagine living in a society in which people exist totally by themselves, unable to share any of themselves with other human beings? Even in an advanced technological society such as ours, there is still a need for person-to-person communication for effective functioning (Fig. 6-1).

"Communication establishes a sense of commonness with another and permits the sharing of information, signals, or messages in the form of ideas and feelings" (Murray & Zentner, 1985, p. 71). To the beginning helper this definition should present a new meaning of a familiar term. Most of us have given thought to the word communication and we would generally agree that to communicate is to impart or share some type of information with another person. The key words in the above definition are: "establishing a sense of commoness." Communication can only occur when both the sender and the receiver have a common understanding of the sender's message. For the purpose of this discussion, the sender is the person transmitting the message, and the receiver is the person for whom the message is intended. Communication is a continuous process that involves both verbal and nonverbal messages. A successful communication occurs when the idea, thought, or message is "conveyed to and understood by another person" (Lewis, 1973, p. 9).

In theory the communication process is quite simple. Note the following diagram:

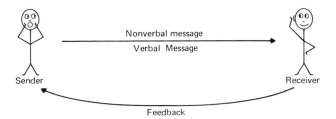

The sender is the person responsible for initiating the communication process. The sender attempts to relate effectively to the receiver by the use of nonverbal and/or verbal techniques. The receiver is responsible for interpreting the message and confirming to the sender that the message is understood. The receiver accomplishes this by giving some type of feedback to the sender that indicates that the message has been interpreted correctly, or if not correctly interpreted, at least heard. There are two types of feedback: direct feedback, in which the receiver understands the message and conveys this information either verbally or nonverbally to the sender, and indirect feedback, in which the receiver knows there is a message being sent but is unclear as to its meaning. Note the following example:

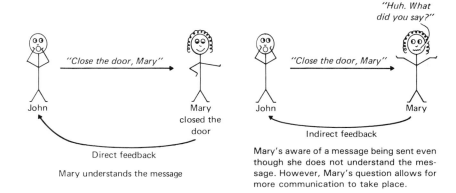

Since this is a cyclic process and must include feedback to be completed, any communication without feedback is ineffective.

In theory, this process seems reasonable and easy to accomplish successfully. However, in all communication interactions, there are always distractors present that can inhibit an effective communication pattern.

Distractors are stimuli which interfere with the communication process. Distractors are either weak or strong. Intense distractors have inhibiting effects upon the communication process. Since we do not live in a vacuum, almost all communication processes have distractors. In other words, there are few, if any, interactions that proceed like this:

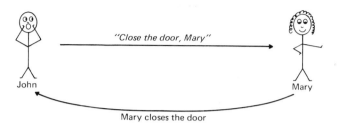

Distractors arise from the sender, the receiver, and the environment and can interfere at any point during the communication process. In all communication processes there are two phases:

- Phase I: This phase occurs during the period of time in which the sender transmits the message to the receiver.
- Phase II: This phase occurs during the period of time in which the receiver acknowledges the message being sent and gives some type of feedback to the sender.

As stated earlier, distractors can occur at any point during the communication process. The following diagram and explanation clarifies for the helper exactly what is meant by distractors that impede communication.

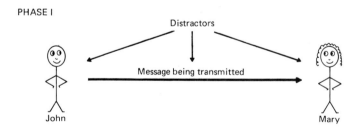

It is important to note that distractors can occur at any point during this process and often are multiple in number. Fortunately, most distractors are mild and do not have inhibiting effects upon the communication process. Distractors often arise from the sender in the form of accent, dress, or voice tone. Usually the receiver is quickly alerted to unusual accents or soft-spoken people and listens more intently to what is being said. However, most of us can remember a time when we have become so engrossed in the sender's personal appearance that we neglected to listen to the message being sent. Fortunately, this situation does not happen too often, and it is easy to remedy.

The environment is usually replete with distractors. Such stimuli as loud music, hot weather, colorful walls, or dogs howling influence the interaction and, depending on the number of distractors and their intensity, may inhibit the communication process. If the environment is too noisy, the message cannot be heard and there is a break in the process. Often the communication process fails because of stimuli influencing the receiver. If the receiver becomes preoccupied with personal matters (such as the college student who fails a final exam), it is often difficult or impossible for the receiver to listen to the message. This same situation is true of a patient who has just been diagnosed as having a dreadful disease. The patient is often unable to hear anything the doctor says after hearing the diagnosis.

PHASE II

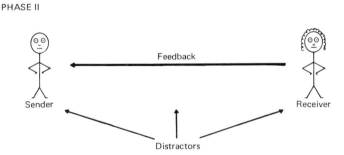

Phase II is similar to Phase I in that distractors continue to arise from the receiver, environment, or sender.

Even though a receiver may hear the message, the subsequent action may not be appropriate. The receiver can easily forget about a message because there are so many other stimuli that influence the situation. Note the following example:

> Marsha calls Susan on the phone. Carol answers and states that Susan will be back at 8 P.M. Marsha asks Carol to have Susan call her the moment she comes home, as she has some important news for her. Carol says, "Sure, I'll have her call the moment she walks in the door." Carol has obviously heard Marsha's message; however, she becomes extremely busy studying for an exam and forgets to tell Susan about the call.

The environment, as in Phase I, can be laden with distractors which, if intense in nature, can inhibit the return of a message. Loud noises such as cars backfiring or radios blasting can interfere with the sender's ability to hear the feedback being sent by the receiver. The sender may interfere in the communication process by sending out a particular message in the hope of getting a particular response and may not hear the actual response given. Note what happens to Jason in the following example:

Jason, who is 6 years old, asks his mother to take him to his friend David's house after school. His mother says that she will be glad to take him, if David's mother calls to invite Jason. Jason becomes excited and begins to plan which toys he will take to David's house.

Jason has heard only part of his mother's response—namely, the part he wanted to hear. He seems to be oblivious to the conditional phrase "if David's mother calls."

In most cases people can overcome the distractors and respond to the sender in an appropriate fashion. As a beginning helper, you must examine the type of feedback the receiver is giving and evaluate whether or not the receiver understands your message. Feedback is not always a verbal response and, therefore, you must begin to look at the more subtle behavior of your client. Note the following examples:

Karen and Sharon are planning a surprise party for Betty. Betty enters the room, and Karen inadvertently mentions the party. Sharon, however, looks at her quite sternly and Karen responds by saying that she is going to a party for her cousin.

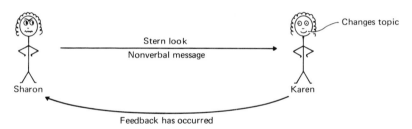

Karen has responded appropriately to Sharon's nonverbal cues, and communication has occurred! Consider this situation:

On the first day of class the teacher mentions that there will be a weekly quiz every Friday, beginning the very first week of class. The teacher says nothing more about the quiz, and over half of the class fails the first quiz. Most of the students who failed claimed they did not hear the announcement about the quizzes.

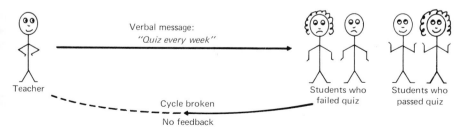

What happened? Can you identify some possible distractors in this situation?

Verbal and nonverbal feedback do not always harmonize. Consider the following:

Kathy and Toni are having a discussion about school. Kathy states that everything is going well but appears very jittery and nervous. Toni notes that Kathy is smoking continuously and tapping her fingers on the desk. Toni responds to Kathy by commenting on her nonverbal message rather than her verbal message.

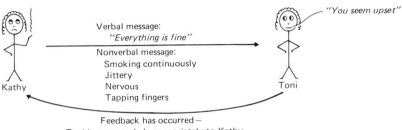

Feedback has occurred —
Toni has responded appropriately to Kathy

This is a bit more complex than the previous examples. It is important to recognize that the helper is in the receiver's position and responsible for giving feedback, not initiating a message. The helper must learn to be flexible, as it is expected that the helper change roles from sender to receiver as the need arises. Thus, being in the position of receiver does not in any way change the helper's position of being responsible to the client. Also, it is important to note that, when verbal and nonverbal messages that do not agree are sent at the same time, the helper must learn to identify the true message. (This latter concept will be discussed later in this chapter.)

VERBAL COMMUNICATION

Since messages are sent in three ways—verbally, nonverbally, or in writing—it is vital for us to examine all three. Let us begin by examining verbal communication.

We usually associate verbal communication with the spoken word. Verbal communication "represents only a small segment of total human communications" (Sundeen, Stuart, Rankin, & Cohen, 1985, p. 95). However, communication often fails because the sender and the receiver do not have a common understanding of the spoken words used during the interaction. This may be because of a language difference (Spanish, English, etc.) or because of a difference in meaning or interpretation of a given word or phrase. Verbal messages may need to be repeated more than once and supplemented with other means of communication, such as pictures or the written word (Johnson, 1972, p. 66). Refer back to the example of the teacher giving directions on the first day of class. Since the teacher's quiz schedule was only mentioned once, the results of not repeating this important information to the class were disastrous. Often distractors arising from either the environment or the receiver alter the receiver's ability to hear the actual message being sent. It is not unusual to hear students deny vehemently that they were told, yet the teacher can document when and how the students were told this information. It might have been helpful for the teacher to repeat this information on another day and to write the date of the first quiz on the blackboard.

Messages also should be as clear and specific as possible. Particular attention should be given to clarification of words or ideas that are being transmitted to the receiver. It is the sender's function to make sure the receiver understands the spoken words of the conversation. "Words can be interpreted in many different ways. And of course this is the basis for many misunderstandings" (Adler & Towne, 1981, p. 300).

> *Dr. Jessup:*   I'm sending you for a test tomorrow. The purpose of the test is to help diagnose your gall bladder disease. Don't worry about it—it is a painless test.
>
> *Mrs. Soars:*   [*After the doctor has left*] I have to go for another test. I'm so afraid. I always have pain when I have tests.

Obviously, the word "test" has a very different meaning to the doctor and to the patient. After talking with Mrs. Soars, you realize that she associates tests with painful procedures such as drawing blood or taking biopsies. Her doctor, however, is talking about a diagnostic x-ray, which is virtually a painless procedure. In discussing the test with the patient, the doctor neglects to observe whether or not the word "test" is understood. A thoughtful helper can assist in clearing up this confusion by explaining to Mrs. Soars what the physician meant by the term "test."

It is important to remember that words are symbols and do not have the same meaning for everyone. It is fundamental to any communication process to use words that have a mutual meaning to those involved. Note the following example:

> Timmy, aged 3, has a bad cold and has been coughing all day long. When he enters the room to ask his mom for a drink, the following exchange occurs:
>
> *Timmy:*   Mommy, Mommy, my voice is funny. Listen . . .
> *Mother:*   Gee, Timmy, I think you have a frog in your throat.
> *Timmy:*   [*His eyes widen*] No, I don't.
> *Mother:*   Not a real frog—it's a word that means you have a bad cold that makes the inside of your throat bigger and you sound like a frog when he croaks.

The mother has noted Timmy's literal interpretation of the phrase "frog in your throat" and has responded appropriately to clarify any confusion Timmy might have. "The denotative meaning of a word refers to some concrete description of the word" (Sundeen et al., 1981, p. 80). In this case, the child understands the word "frog" to mean a small animal. However, his mother has attached a connotative meaning to this word and understands the term "frog in your throat" to mean a scratchy throat. "The personalized or connotative meaning varies with past experiences, present frame of reference, and other internal variables" (Sundeen et al., 1985, p. 97).

As professional helpers, you will quickly learn that verbal communication takes place at several levels, and you must be able to adapt quickly to each level. Clients, generally, require one form of language: direct, clear, and concise. Depending upon the cognitive abilities of the client, vocabulary can be simple or complex. Helpers must always be careful that they are not "talking down" to clients.

> Patrick Hart is a lively, 75-year-old resident in a home for the elderly. About 6 weeks ago he fractured his hip and since that time has been seeing a physical therapist for biweekly sessions. Mr. Lovett, the therapist, is amazed at Patrick's ability to crutch walk and his understanding of bone healing. Mr. Hart listens intently to all explanations and consistently demonstrates ability to follow the therapist's directions. Mr. Lovett is clear about explaining exercises, using simple but correct medical terminology. He also demonstrates each activity along with discussing what is expected of Mr. Hart.

It is important that we learn to use verbal communication effectively, as this form of communication is under our conscious control. It is important that we learn to speak in clear, concise terms and to validate the receiver's understanding in order to prevent confusion.

NONVERBAL COMMUNICATION

"Nonverbal communication is the way in which human beings influence each other without words—the way in which man expresses himself through a silent language and makes an impression on others" (Collins, 1977, p. 62). Our nonverbal behavior is often more revealing of our true feelings than our verbal behavior. Our verbal behavior is much more deliberate. We can control our verbal responses, thus hiding our true feelings. Nonverbal communication is usually spontaneous. Since our nonverbal behavior is often unplanned, we respond in an honest fashion—we are less apt to "play games" and try to fool others (Fig. 6–2).

Body motion or body language is one of the most common ways we communicate nonverbally with others. Those of us who stand up straight with our heads held high convey a message of self-confidence, while those of us who walk with slumped shoulders and eyes grazing the ground convey a less than confident image. Often, when the use of verbal channels of communication are not practical, gestures that have a common understanding to everyone can replace words (Knapp, 1978) (Fig. 6–3).

The politician who waves to the crowd as he rides by in a parade is one example of how communication can occur without verbalization. The "A-OK" sign and the "peace" sign are two common gestures which are familiar to many of us (Knapp, 1978). Sometimes when we communicate verbally we use nonverbal communication to emphasize our verbal message. When explaining the size of an object, we often use gestures to help give the listener a more accurate idea of the actual size. When we are frustrated, we may raise our hands in the air to help demonstrate our helplessness in this situation. The mother who scolds her child for breaking a dish may point a finger to the dish as well as verbally reprimand the child.

Nonverbal messages are often complex and it takes a great deal of practice to decipher their meanings accurately. Nonverbal messages can be conveyed in several ways—gestures, silence, or touch. All three can be quite significant, and it is vitally important that the beginning helper study all communication interactions on both their verbal and nonverbal levels. Nonverbal behavior must always be examined concurrently with verbal behavior. Often the nonverbal behavior of the client may give the helper an idea of what message the client is really sending, even though the verbal message may be distinctly opposite to the nonverbal one. Consider the following examples:

Gloria and Frank have been dating steadily for two years. She is anxious to get married and they have talked about it, but have no definite plans and are not engaged. It is Gloria's birthday, and Frank has taken her out to dinner and is about to give her a present.

Frank: [Smiling] Would you like to open your gift now?

Gloria: [Smiling] Sure.

Frank: [Putting a small jewelry box on the table and looking very serious] I hope you like it.

Gloria: [Opening her eyes quite wide and practically gasping in astonishment as she begins to open it] Oh Frank, you shouldn't have.

Frank: I picked it out myself; maybe I should have had you help me.

Gloria: [Opening the box and gazing at large opal earrings, she remains silent for awhile] Thank you. [Her enthusiastic mood has become quite somber]

Frank: Don't you like them?

Gloria: They are beautiful; of course I like them. [Followed by a long silent pause]

Frank: You don't seem happy.

In this example, Gloria is trying to convey verbally that she is pleased with earrings, even though they are not what she expected. However, her nonverbal message of disappointment seems to be overriding her verbal message.

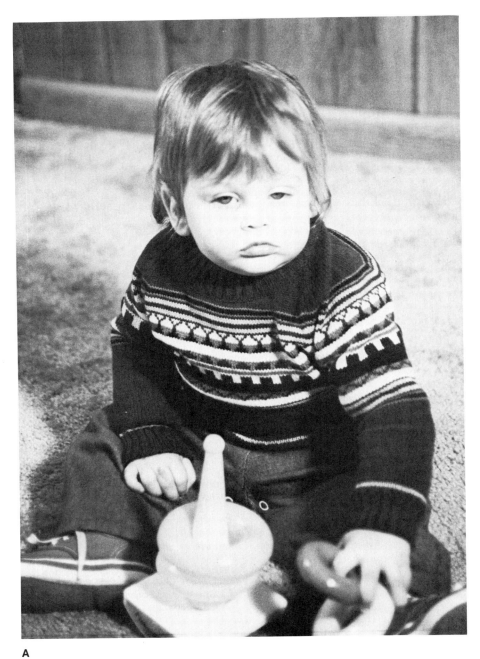

A

Figure 6-2. Can you identify the nonverbal messages in each of these pictures?

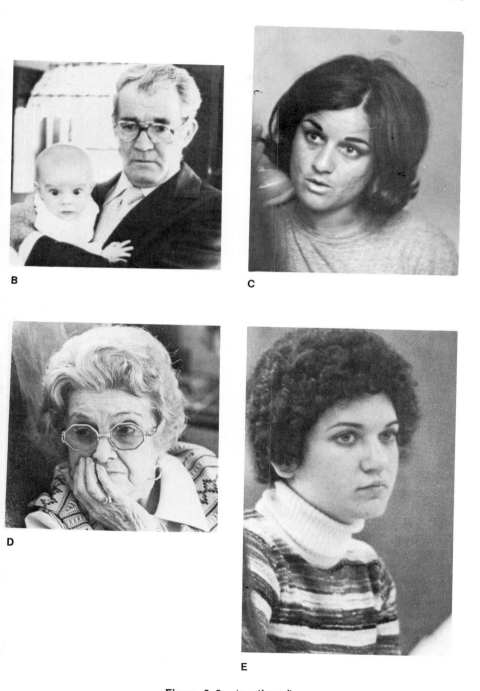

B

C

D

E

Figure 6-2. (continued)

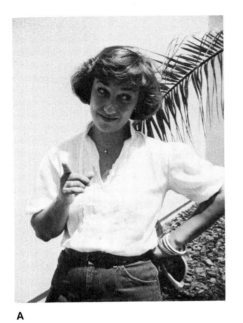

A

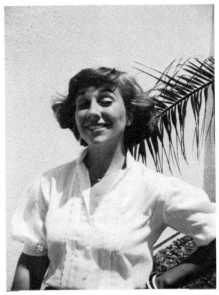

B

C

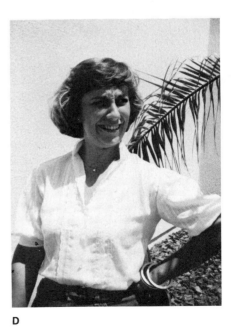

D

Figure 6-3. Ideas can be communicated through body language.
(Photo credit to Peggy Haggerty.)

Her entire affect has changed—her excitement has turned to disappointment. There are long periods of silence during the conversation, which in this instance convey a nonverbal message of disappointment to Frank. Facial expressions are most revealing, and it is impossible for Gloria to disguise her true feelings.

> The human body or parts thereof have been considered to symbolize characteristics of the soul, the mood, or the temperament of the person. From the beginning of recorded history, men have been guided in their judgments by the observation of facial expression. (Reusch & Kees, 1966, p. 39)

Martha and Donna are graduate students in a counseling program. It is the end of the semester and Donna, an honor student, is preparing for comprehensive examinations. At this moment, she is talking to Martha about her upcoming exams.

Donna: [*Looking tired and discouraged*] I think I am going to fail. I just don't have enough time to finish my course work and to prepare for comps. [*Looking at the floor*]

Martha: [*Shaking her head in agreement*] You feel you are going to fail comps . . .

Donna: [*Looking up rather quickly*] I don't really think I'll fail. I just have so much to do.

Martha: It is scary, and it would be a shame to flunk out at this point in the game.

In this particular situation, Donna's initial verbal communication is quite contrary to what she truly believes. Surely an honor student does not really need to have a deep concern about failing. However, Donna may be feeling overwhelming pressure to complete her end of the semester papers as well as comprehensive exams. Martha is only listening to the verbal context of the situation; she is not attempting to delve into the real problem. Even though her technique of repeating what Donna has stated is appropriate, it does not help to get to the real issue of how Donna is feeling.

Consider the following:

Donna: [*Looking tired and discouraged*] I think I'm going to fail. I just don't have enough time to finish my course work and to prepare for comps. [*Looking at the floor*]

Martha: Donna, you look so tired—you have really been working so hard.

Donna: [*Sighing*] I have—I have been studying until all hours of the morning and sleeping in short naps.

Martha: Sounds like you really need a good night's rest.

Donna: [*Nodding in agreement*] I do. I think if I have about 10 hours' sleep, I'll be more refreshed and I'll get more work done.

In this instance, Martha picked up on Donna's physical appearance and communicated to Donna in response to her nonverbal rather than verbal behavior. In the first situation, Martha focused only on the aspects of the verbal interaction and did not respond to the total situation.

The following is an example in which the sender and the receiver relate effectively without any verbal communication:

> Mr. Sands is a freshman biology teacher, and Jenny is a good student who is always prepared for class. Mr. Sands notes on this particular day that Jenny looks unusually tired, and whenever he asks the class questions, she looks at the floor, avoiding any eye-to-eye contact with him. Because of her nonverbal behavior, he decides not to question her directly. She is saying to him, without using any form of verbal communication, that she does not want to participate today. Mr. Sands demonstrates his concern for Jenny by "hearing" her message and respecting her temporary detachment from the discussion.

Although in the examples given, the nonverbal cues are easily identifiable, in real life these cues are often somewhat obscure. Therefore, it is important that the beginning helper fully develop and use all of the senses in order to accurately assess each situation.

OBSERVATION AND PERCEPTION

Those of us engaged in helping professions are constantly being asked to observe people and the surrounding environment. Until now, you probably have been using your eyes to do most of your observing. Most of us tend to rely heavily on our sense of sight when making observations, forgetting how helpful our senses of sound, touch, and smell can be. Later in this chapter the usefulness of all four of these senses will be discussed.

Before we can learn how to make accurate observations, we must have a clear understanding of the concept of observation. Observation is a systematic, nonjudgmental process that cannot be accomplished in a haphazard fashion. To do so would be gross negligence on the part of the person responsible for making the observations. The main aim of the helping person when observing other people is to "monitor the reactions of the receiver to the words or gestures of the sender and to determine if in fact the receiver did receive the correct message" (Hein, 1973, p. 151). The main aim of the helping person when observing the environment is to describe the situation accurately in a nonbiased manner.

Our ability to observe either people or situations depends upon our ability to differentiate observations from perceptions. An observation is a factual report, while a perception is the "personal interpretation of observations" (Murray & Zentner, 1985, p. 79). Our ability to access the client and the situation accurately correlates with our ability to make nonjudgmental observations. Perceptions, whether they be true or not, have a definite sense of reality about them. Perceptions of events vary from person to person and are dependent upon that which the person is prepared for or wishes to see (Murray & Zentner, 1985). Note the following example:

> Ron and Gary are college seniors majoring in accounting. Their final grades have just been received in the mail and, together, they open them. Gary has received a "C" in Accounting IV and Ron has received an "A."
>
> Gary: [*Excitedly*] Hey, I got a "C" in Accounting IV.
> Ron: A "C"! Gee, that's too bad.
> Gary: Too bad . . . I'm glad I passed.
> Ron: Oh! It's just that graduate schools are only accepting students with "B" or better averages.

In this situation, Ron is responding to Gary's news of a "C" grade by allowing his feelings about the grade to enter into the interaction. Ron perceives the "C" to mean a closed door to graduate school admission. Gary is happy about the fact that he passed—his perceptions are very different from Ron's. Since perceptions of the same situation can markedly differ from one person to the next, it is important that the helper at least be aware of these differences. If a "C" is a cause of celebration, it is important that the helper recognize this. The helper must begin by responding to what is real for the client. If the client's sense of reality is distorted, then the helper must attempt to correct the distortion. Note the following example:

> Carol is an attractive 25-year-old secretary. She is 5 ft. 4 in. tall and weighs 110 lbs. As a child, Carol was overweight, and she continues to think of herself as obese. Claudia is presently trying to talk Carol into buying a two-piece bathing suit.
>
> Claudia: You could at least try on a two-piece suit.
> Carol: I'm too fat—all my bulges will show!
> Claudia: Fat! You're skin and bones. Come on, try one on.
> Carol: You'll just say how awful I look.
> Claudia: Just try one on—I'll refrain from all negative comments.
> Carol: OK.

Later, when Carol models the suit, two salesgirls comment on how attractive she looks. Carol is pleased with her appearance and buys the suit.

In real life, Carol's perception of herself as being obese would not be this simple to remedy. However, by trying on the two-piece suit and by having people praise her appearance, Carol is forced to look more objectively into the mirror. Her distorted viewpoint can now be changed, as she has some concrete evidence to support Claudia's comments about her weight.

Our perceptions should enhance our observations. Remember, in any situation that you are asked to observe, you must be consciously aware of what you are doing. Observation is a planned activity in which you utilize your senses to help you to collect data. Since it is impractical to observe without interpreting, it is extremely important that you practice interpreting in a nonbiased fashion. As your skill in observing increases, your perceptions will become more accurate. You must learn to look at the situation through the client's eyes and not to burden the client with your thoughts and feelings.

As stated earlier, the use of the senses helps us to make more accurate observations. It is important for you to remember that the sense of sight, smell, sound, and touch can be used together to help you make an accurate observation. You may find that particular situations call upon one sense more than another. It is your responsibility to choose the appropriate method—to choose the method or methods that will help you to collect the most data.

Sight

The sense of sight is, perhaps, the most common sense we use when making observations. When using this sense, the observer often notes only one particular portion of the situation, namely, the part that is of interest to him or her. If the observer has certain preconceived notions or perceptions of a situation, the observation being made may be influenced. The observer uses a personal set of values and transposes these into the situation, thus clouding the issue. Once these preconceived notions are recognized, the observer can consciously work at not letting them interfere with observations. Training the eyes to encompass the entire situation then becomes the major task of the observer. Note the following exercise:

Exercise 1

The purpose of this exercise is to help you to enhance your observational skills. Please do exercise 1 now before continuing to read this chapter.

Look at the picture. What do you see? Write down your observations.

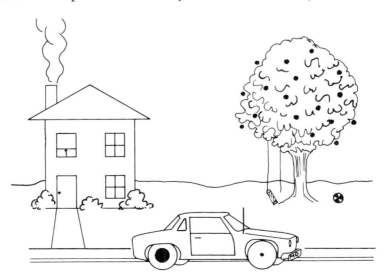

Did you accurately describe each detail (i.e., in this picture there is smoke coming from the chimney; there is a broken swing; one window shade is down; there is fruit on the tree; one hubcap is missing; a ball is on the grass; the car has an antenna and the initials "MD"; there is a sidewalk along the curb). If so, you have developed some sound, value-free, observation skills.

If, however, you made up a little story about a child falling from a swing, hurt, with a doctor coming to the rescue then you are quite creative but need to develop some skill in reporting *only* what you see.

Exercise 2 is designed to help you continue practicing your observational skills. Please complete Exercise 2 now.

Exercise 2

Look around the room. Pick one person you find interesting. Describe what you see by writing down your comments. Do this now before reading on.
Comments such as:

- wearing blue shirt
- brown eyes
- hair shoulder length   } are value free.
- tapping fingers
- biting fingernails

- long hair
- looks tired
- sloppy dresser   } are value laden.
- pretty eyes
- anxiously pacing

When doing this exercise, you may have focused on objective value-free observations or nonobjective value-laden observations. Value-laden statements are a matter of opinion and are not necessarily true. You should avoid these. Practice daily observing both people and the environment. Note the kinds of things you observe; i.e., do you tend to observe what the person is doing or the physical characteristics of that person? Try to combine your observations so that you learn to watch both. Be consciously aware of physical properties and physical activities. Report all of what you observe. Remember, "an observation is a factual report of something in our physical world" (Hein, 1973, p. 152).

Listening

Another important skill for the helper to learn is the art of listening attentively. Listening is an active process involving more than the mere stimulation of nerve endings that allow us to hear. Listening is a purposeful activity and involves the use of the eyes as well as the ears. According to Lewis, "effective listening requires three ingredients: discipline, concentration, and comprehension" (Lewis, 1973, p. 15). Most of us are more comfortable talking than listening. Attentive listening is a skill that requires much practice. We need to discipline ourselves to practice this skill routinely, for without it, we lose much of our ability to help others. Listening requires all of our concentration. If our mind begins to wander, we risk not hearing all of what the client has to say. If we listen attentively, hearing all the words but not understanding the message, something has gone wrong. "Comprehension involves the attempt to understand and grasp the true idea or meaning of what is heard" (Lewis, 1973, p. 37). Many of us selectively listen—we hear only that which we wish to hear. If this occurs, we are unable to interpret the client's total message and, thus, we have limited comprehension of what is being said. Note the following example:

> Dot and Dan have a dinner date. They are to meet at 6 P.M. Dan tells Dot to wait in front of the Redford Bank at North Main Street. Upon hearing the words "Redford Bank," Dot, who is in a hurry, automatically assumes Dan means the branch located on Providence Street, and does not bother to listen to the entire message. At 6 P.M. they are both waiting for each other, but Dot is not in the right place.

Dot has failed to hear the entire message because she has not used good listening skills. She heard only that portion of the message that was of interest to her. She has not understood Dan's total message and is unable to follow through with their plans. Because Dot was in a hurry, she did not take the time to concentrate on the conversation and to listen carefully to the directions.

All of us know how to listen, or at least we think we do. However, most of us need to practice listening and to think consciously about the process as we engage in it. The following three principles should help us to prepare for listening situations.

- *Always listen attentively.* If you are trying to listen to someone, you must consciously ignore your own personal circumstances and distracting environmental influences. The client deserves your full attention. Make sure both of you are comfortable and that you are both situated in such a way that eye-to-eye contact is facilitated.
- *Listen for repetition of key words or themes in the conversation.* Many beginning helpers fear they will miss the point the client is trying to make because at first they are not able to decipher what is important and what is not. Most clients are persistent people who have a need to talk about their problems. Generally, they repeat that which is important to them several times during a conversation.
- *Listen completely.* Do not try to finish phrases or sentences for the client. Begin to examine your own listening habits. Do you wait for

people to finish talking, or do you interrupt and complete sentences for them? Try to listen to what is being said, not to what you want to hear.

Touch

A nonverbal skill that can be very effective when helping people is the use of touch. Researchers frequently discuss the importance of tactile stimulation for normal growth and development of the infant. Montague (1971) found that tactile stimulation during infancy and childhood is necessary for normal growth and development. The infant who receives more caressing and cuddling seems to thrive in his or her environment, as compared to the child from whom tactile stimulation is withheld.

"Touch is a crucial aspect of most human relationships. It plays a part in giving encouragement, expressing tenderness, showing emotional support, and many other things" (Knapp, 1978, p. 243). Touch can communicate feelings between people who care about one another, when words would fail (Murray & Zentner, 1985, p. 87). Touch is not a skill that most of us use automatically. We have the tendency to refrain from employing this skill because of all the taboos on touching in our culture. While we commonly hold, cuddle, and touch infants, as the child grows and reaches adolescence, touch is often restricted with increasing age, and physical contact becomes much more limited, emotional, and value laden (Fig. 6-4). In some households physical contact may be prohibited and viewed as sexual rather than as an expression of caring. For these reasons the helper may find that the therapeutic use of touch may not be appropriate for all clients. In fact, the use of this technique may also not be appropriate for the helper. If the helper feels uncomfortable with the physical use of touch, it is not an appropriate helping technique for that helper. How do you know if a technique does not fit? If you are hesitant to hold someone who is crying or if you feel foolish holding the hand of another during the helping situation, these techniques probably are not working for you. Remember, clients sense your reluctance to communicate in this fashion and recognize that you are not being genuine. However, if you feel these techniques could be helpful, you certainly can practice perfecting them.

To do this, begin to note consciously how often you use physical contact in your day-to-day communication. For example, do you ever put your arm around a friend while talking? Do you play contact sports? Do you frequently kiss or hug family members?

Next, note how you respond to physical contact. Does it make you squirm or feel uncomfortable? Does it make you feel calm and secure? Does it make you feel that someone cares about you?

"To be able to touch another physically, emotionally, mentally, or socially—is a distinct art" (Obrien, 1978, p. 100). Although you may not be

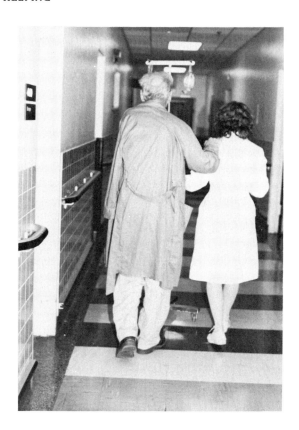

Figure 6-4. Clients use touch, as well as helpers. (*Photo credit to Peggy Haggerty.*)

using touch gracefully in a therapeutic situation, if you feel positively about its benefits, you should consider practicing until you perfect the skill. As with all skills, at first touching may seem awkward, artificial, or phony. Give yourself time—eventually you will find you are using touch without even realizing it.

There are some clients who respond positively to touch and some who do not. The helper must learn to judge when this technique will be effective and respond accordingly. Even though the helper's attitude about touch can be changed, sometimes the client's feelings cannot. Some, not all, clients may view this technique as offensive, uncomfortable, or sexual in nature. It is best to call upon other techniques to help these clients. Occasionally a client may reach out and touch, or hold, the helper. If the helper is uncomfortable about this, it is best to get out of the situation as gracefully as possible. Discussing one's uncomfortableness might be a possibility in some relationships. In some situations where the client and the helper are at opposite poles on their use and comfortableness of touch, referral to another helper is the best solution.

Even after making a careful assessment of the client, the helper may wrongly decide to use touch. Consider Mary, an 18-year-old college student enrolled in a group communications course:

> During the semester Mary has discussed with the class her Portuguese background, her love of her grandmother, and her family life-style. The semester is almost finished, and Mary asks to meet with the teacher. She is crying and obviously very upset.
>
> *Teacher:* Come in, Mary, and sit down.
>
> *Mary:* [*Sobbing*] Thank you—I just needed to talk to someone.
>
> *Teacher:* You seem upset—has something happened?
>
> *Mary:* My grandmother is dying—it's just a matter of time! [*Sobbing*]
>
> *Teacher:* [*Extends her hand over Mary's*] I'm so sorry to hear that.
>
> *Mary:* [*Immediately moves her hand away—continues to sob*]
>
> *Teacher:* This must be very difficult for you; I know how much you loved her. [*Withholds the use of touch—looks directly at Mary*]
>
> *Mary:* It's so hard to believe—I knew this would happen some day but it is still hard to believe.

In this situation, the teacher thought she knew which technique would be most effective with Mary. After assessing Mary's cultural background and her verbal participation in the classroom, the teacher felt the use of touch would be comforting in this situation. To her surprise, the teacher found that Mary rejected this intervention, and the teacher appropriately changed her approach.

If both the client and the helper are comfortable with the use of touch as a therapeutic, nonverbal technique, it can have a very soothing and calming effect upon the client. Unfortunately, the use of touch becomes somewhat of a lost art as the client grows older. Although we commonly use touch to comfort infants and young children, we tend not to use this technique with older clients. This is an unfortunate situation because we know that the elderly, also, need physical affection. Those people who are receptive to its use find the warm touch of a caring person helps them to feel secure. It is as if the helper, through the therapeutic use of touch, is able to impart some of his inner strength to the client (Jourard, 1971).

Smell

One of the least-used senses is that of smell. Most helpers do not rely upon the olfactory sense when engaging in therapeutic situations. "The receptors for smell are easily fatigued after several minutes of continuous stimulation by a specific odor" (Lewis, 1973, p. 49). This accounts for part of the reason why helpers are not tuned into using this sense. Those people working in hospitals soon become accustomed to the strange odors and are unaware of their offensiveness to clients. Another reason why this sense is often ignored relates to the fact that most people use their ability to smell to make negative observations. Our society is quite conscious of "bad breath" and "body odor," and often helpers have little practice in distinguishing pleasanter odors.

Helpers must practice observing the pleasant and unpleasant scents in our environment. The mother of an infant soon becomes aware of the offensive odors of fecal elimination and quickly remedies the problem. An adolescent's mother notes changes in body odor and encourages the youth to begin using a deodorant. These are some simple examples of the way in which helpers usually utilize their olfactory sense.

How can a helper utilize the olfactory sense to help assess the client's behavior? Remember, since the sense of smell is quickly lost, all olfactory observations should be made when first seeing the client. Practice observing pleasant odors. When you enter someone's home, note the pleasant smell of fresh-baked bread. Note the client's choice of perfume and after-shave lotion. These can be very important.

When assessing the client's health status and adaptation to the environment, you might possibly develop a clue to the client's overall general hygienic practices by noting a clean, fresh body odor. On the other hand, you may note that the perfume is acting as an unsuccessful cover-up for poor hygienic practices. You may also note changes in the client's well-being by being cognizant that your client, who was once slovenly, is now neatly dressed and always smells good. This may be an indication that the client is feeling better about him- or herself.

The helper must become cognizant of personal reactions to odors, especially unpleasant ones. A hospitalized patient with cancer may be totally helpless in controlling the offensive odors caused by deteriorating body tissue. If a nurse, social worker, or doctor facially expresses a dislike of this odor, the patient may interpret this to mean, "I don't like you because you smell funny." Therefore, it is "more helpful to the patient to indicate verbally that you know the odor must be distressful to him" (Lewis, 1973, p. 51). In making this type of comment, it brings the situation out in the open and allows the patient a chance to talk about feelings relating to the unpleasant odor—an almost unheard-of subject of conversation in our society. Obviously, comments of this nature must be made in a tactful manner. Once the client and helper have developed a more trusting relationship, the client may be more willing to discuss personal feelings about the unpleasant odor.

The refinement of our ability to perceive and observe others will help us in our day-to-day interactions with clients. The beginning helper must make a conscious effort to practice utilizing these observational skills in daily life. The ability to make concrete, accurate, and nonjudgmental observations is not innate—the helper needs to develop this skill. The more proficient he or she becomes in using the senses, the more skill and expertise the helper brings to a professional situation.

WRITTEN COMMUNICATION

In addition to making nonbiased observations and communicating clearly, professional helpers have a further responsibility: to document in writing their encounters with clients.

Although the nature of this documentation may vary from profession to profession, the basic principles are the same. All helpers must first learn to consider written documentation as an important part of the communication process and to assume responsibility for accurate, prompt documentation of events that have occurred. Many written records, such as nurses' notes, are legal documents and, thus, subject to the scrutiny of the courts.

Professional helpers must familiarize themselves with the method of record keeping for their profession. Members of the health professions often keep "running notes" or logs that inform the reader of the date and time of an event, as well as what occurred during that observation period. These notes need not be long or involved. However, it is necessary that notes be accurate and inclusive. Compare the following notes written by a physical therapist:

10 A.M.	Leg lift exercises done, tolerated poorly.
10 A.M.	Leg lift exercises—able to lift ⓇЁ leg 60° without complaining of pain. Moved Ⓛ leg 30°, complained of sharp pain in the gluteal muscle.

Observe that the second note is far more comprehensive, indicating to the reader exactly where the pain was, how much movement of the legs was accomplished, and what the differences were between the right and left leg. Statements like "tolerated poorly" are too general and subjective. These types of statements have different meanings to each of us; thus, there is no universal agreement about the word "poorly." Each of us, however, has an understanding of 30° and sharp pain in the gluteal muscle. Professional helpers must strive for specificity.

Frequently, the purpose of written communication is to relay directions or specific information to clients, to their families, and/or to other professional helpers. It is necessary that these messages be clear and concise, or the recipients of them will not understand their meaning. Note the following example of Susan Lang, the principal of Brookfield High School:

> Every year in April Susan Lang writes work evaluations for her faculty. This year she is in a hurry and tries to condense her workload. She decides that Mrs. Ames, Ms. Hirchl, and Ms. Waldorf are all contributing in a similar manner and, therefore, she writes to each of them, "It is expected because of your long-standing positions on this faculty that you will assume a leadership role, and in the coming year your contributions to the development of our curriculum will continue to increase and be productive."

In talking to each of the three teachers who received this message, it becomes clear to Susan Lang that she has made a dreadful mistake. Mrs. Ames thinks that the note is a vote of confidence for a job well done. Ms. Hirchl is angry, feeling the evaluation should address what was done during this year, not what should occur next year. Ms. Waldorf is upset with herself, feeling that the note is saying that she needs to be producing more.

Needless to say, Susan Lang has to communicate more effectively. She has written such a general statement that it is subject to several interpretations. A little forethought would have saved many of the misunderstandings that occurred once the note had been sent.

Finally, written commmunication must be grammatically correct. Obviously, a less formal, handwritten message need not be as exact as more formal communications. However, the more exact you are, the easier it is for you to share your thoughts and observations in writing. Remember, other people evaluate your performance, in part, by the way in which you write. To gain their respect, you need to spell, structure sentences, and punctuate correctly. Professional helpers have a responsibility first to objectively observe and then to record precisely that which they have observed.

IMPORTANT REMINDERS

1. Communication establishes a sense of commonness in which we share information, ideas, and feelings with another person(s).
2. Communication is a cyclic process, and this cycle must contain feedback for the process to occur.
3. Distractors are common to all communication processes and may be so intense that they have an inhibiting effect upon the interaction.
4. The sender and the receiver must have a common base for the definition of words. Frequent feedback is helpful in assessing the receiver's understanding of the spoken words.
5. Nonverbal communication is more subtle and more spontaneous than verbal communication. Since we do not consciously control our nonverbal communication, it is more representative of our true feelings.
6. Observation is a systematic, nonjudgmental process involving skillful use of the senses—sight, sound, touch, and smell.
7. The principles of written communication for you as a professional helper are: developing an attitude that values written communication; familiarizing yourself with the documentation processes of your profession; writing grammatically correct, value-free notes that are clear, concise, and accurate.

REFERENCES

Adler, R., & Towne, N. (1981). *Looking out/looking in—Interpersonal communication* (3rd ed.). New York: Holt, Rinehart & Winston.

Collins, M. (1977). *Communication in health care*. St. Louis; C.V. Mosby.

Hein, E. (1973). *Communication in nursing practice*. Boston: Little, Brown.

Johnson, D. (1972). *Reaching out*. Englewood Cliffs, N. J.: Prentice-Hall.

Jourard, S. (1971). *The transparent self*. New York: Van Noal Rand.

Knapp, M. (1978). *Nonverbal communication in human interaction* (2nd ed.). New York: Holt, Rinehart & Winston.

Lewis, G. (1973). *Nurse-patient communication*. Dubuque, Iowa: Brown.

Montague, A. (1971). *Touching: The human significance of skin*. New York: Harper & Row.

Murray, R., & Zentner, J. (1985). *Nursing concepts for health promotion*. Englewood Cliffs, N.J.: Prentice-Hall.

Obrien, M. (1978). *Communications and relationships in nursing*. St. Louis: C. V. Mosby.

Reusch, J., & Kess, W. (1966). *Nonverbal communication*. Los Angeles: University of California Press.

Sundeen, S. J., Stewart, G. W., Rankin, E. D., & Cohen, S. A. (1985). *Nurse–client interaction*. St. Louis: C. V. Mosby.

The best may slip, and the most cautious fall; he's more than mortal that ne'er err'd at all.

John Pomfret

7

Barriers to Effective Communication

Upon completion of the following reading and suggested exercises, the student will be able to:

1. Discuss how sensory overload, noise, deep-rooted philosophical differences, and lack of honesty serve as barriers to effective communication.
2. Name and describe the following barriers to effective communication:
   False reassurance
   Giving advice
   Probing
   Changing the subject
   Minimizing feelings
   Using trite expressions
   Jumping to conclusions
   Inappropriate use of facts
   Interrupting
   Prolonged use of silence
3. Identify the effects of each of these barriers upon the communication process.
4. Analyze the effects of each of these barriers upon the communication process.

DEFINITION OF BARRIERS TO COMMUNICATION

Parry (1968) defines barriers to communication as obstacles that prevent or block the communication process. It is important that you become knowledgeable about these barriers if your intent is to help clients by using a therapeutic process. Although on the surface these barriers may seem exceedingly easy to remedy, you may find that in the real world of practice they are not quite that simple.

Sensory Overload

In an effort to be helpful, you may attempt to give a lot of information to the client, often more information than the client needs.

Have you ever listened to a teacher give a detailed explanation of how to solve a math problem and then left the class not knowing what the teacher was talking about? You need to remember that people can only see, hear, and comprehend so much. Most of us cannot really give our full attention to a task for more than 50 minutes. Sometimes rushing through material or adding on an extra 10 minutes serves only to frustrate rather than to help the client. Being able to pick out the salient facts, repeating important ideas, and asking for feedback to see if the ideas have been received as intended "is far more useful than overloading the client with a lot of extraneous information" (Sundeen, Stuart, Rankin, & Cohen, 1981, p. 98).

Noise

Noise, be it internal or external, is an important factor to consider when attempting to help a client. Internal noises or distractions, such as fatigue, hunger, or stress, must quickly be identified. Although not all of these distractions can be remedied immediately, some can. A good night's sleep or a nutritious meal can do a lot to rejuvenate a client's body and, sometimes, his or her sense of well-being. Helpers need to identify internal noises, as many of these need to be taken care of before a therapeutic process can begin.

External noise is not always possible to control, although it is easier to identify. Loud music, warm temperatures, or dingy, dark rooms may interfere with the process. Interestingly, the client may not find this external noise noxious, especially if he or she is used to it. Often it is the helper, who may be visiting the client's setting, who has difficulty with these stimuli. In the best of all situations, client interviews should be conducted in a "quiet, private, comfortable area to decrease the deleterious effects of environmental noise" (Sundeen et al., 1981, p. 98).

Deep-Rooted Philosophical Differences

You will care for many clients who have value systems and religious beliefs very different from your own. Certainly, you are aware that each person has the inalienable right to his or her beliefs, and that those beliefs must be respected by the helper. On occasion, and this is generally rare, the helper and client come from such diverse philosophical backgrounds that it is impossible for the relationship to grow. Consider the parents who refuse medical treatment for a child because they feel it is "against God's will." Clearly, there are some helpers who would have difficulty withholding treatment; thus, their role with this family must be considered carefully. As a helper, you must begin to gain insight into your philosophical beliefs and be honest about admitting to areas in which you might not be the best person to care for a particular client.

Lack of Honesty

Honesty is a basic element in all trusting encounters. If you believe that trust is inherent in all therapeutic relationships, you will agree that honesty is an essential component of that relationship. Both the client and the helper need to feel secure with the fact that each is being truthful. Consider the following example:

> Carla is an honor student presently participating in a seminar course on death and dying. She has to present and write three papers as part of the course requirements.
> After presenting her first paper, Carla feels somewhat confused—she is not sure she did her best. The teacher, Mr. Bowen, is someone she respects and trusts. She asks the teacher for feedback about her presentation. He tells her the strengths and weaknesses he noted, indicating specific areas in which she can improve. Carla knows that this information will be helpful for the next papers and trusts that the teacher will judge her on her growth, not her past mistakes.

Most clients are looking for the truth, an honest response. Carla wants to improve; she does not expect Mr. Bowen to tell her all was fine. Think about Carla's feelings if Mr. Bowen told her not to worry but then failed her in the course.

If the client and helper are truly engaging in a trusting relationship, the process will be productive. As stated earlier, trust is not an innate characteristic of a relationship—it is an element that evolves—that becomes! In this chapter we will discuss those factors that inhibit the communication process. This chapter is designed to help the student become a better facilitator by avoiding techniques that hinder this process. In the next chapter we will discuss communication skills that help to facilitate the process and to encourage trust.

EFFECTS OF COMMUNICATION BARRIERS ON THE COMMUNICATION PROCESS

It is important to recognize that we are all guilty of using nontherapeutic techniques from time to time. Somehow they seem to "slip out" before we realize what we are saying. An occasional mistake in no way hinders the overall helping process. If anything, it verifies to the client that we are human, that we make mistakes, too! If your relationship with the client is one that is built on trust, it will withstand a few blunders in technique. However, it is crucial that the helper begin to recognize mistakes and the implications of overuse of nontherapeutic communication skills upon the entire process. Thus, an occasional error is expected. The process will continue to grow if trust has been established and if the client feels the helper really cares.

Some nontherapeutic responses occur simply because we are in the habit of using them, with no forethought as to the implications they have upon the total communication process. These nontherapeutic responses can also be termed barriers to effective communication. They are the type of responses that close doors—they do not encourage the client to move and grow in the helping situation. They are inhibitory. They produce stagnation at best and regression at worst.

False Reassurance

There are several approaches that a well-meaning but poorly informed helper might take to inhibit the communication process. Probably one of the most common errors the uninformed helper commits is that of false reassurance. This occurs when the helper in effect tells the client, "Everything will be OK— do not worry." Such statements belittle "the person who feels he has legitimate problems and . . . discourages . . . further expression of feelings and trust" (Murray & Zentner, 1985, p. 102). Consider the following example:

> Joni is a 30-year-old divorcee and mother of twin boys, age 8. She is a secretary who is supporting her family on a limited income of $13,000 per year. She is proud that she has not had to ask for public assistance and that she has been able to make ends meet. On Friday, her boss, Mr. Philips, calls her in his office and tells her she is laid off because the company cannot afford her position. Later that evening, she is discussing the situation with a friend, Nancy.
>
> *Joni:*   I don't know what I'll do. My poor boys.
> *Nancy:* You must feel terrible.
> *Joni:*   It's really discouraging. I've worked so hard.
> *Nancy:* But there are other jobs.
> *Joni:*   Yes, but they are not easy to get, and being laid off doesn't look good on my record.
> *Nancy:* I'm sure everything will be OK.
> *Joni:*   Yeah—I suppose so.

Although Nancy does show a concern for Joni, she has minimized the seriousness of Joni's problems. Her comments relating to other jobs and everything being OK may sound reassuring, but in reality Nancy is not justified in saying these things because she cannot predict what the future will be like. She really has no way of foreseeing that everything in effect will be "OK."

Many of us are guilty of saying to friends, "Don't worry; everything will be all right." Somehow this makes us feel good because we can respond in a reassuring fashion. However, the response is not an honest one, it merely lets us "off the hook." In essence, we are not forced to respond to how the client is really feeling. Nondirectly, we are saying to the client, "Your problem is not that big or that bad." We are not being empathetic. We are not trying to see the problem as the client sees it.

Thus, falsely reassuring will serve to negate the client's feelings and to block communication regarding these feelings (Sundeen, 1985). Joni quickly realizes that Nancy is not going to listen, so she responds somewhat hesitantly, "Yeah, I suppose so," thus closing the door to further discussion of her true feelings. This conversation may continue, but Joni probably will keep agreeing that everything will be OK and will discuss how her boss fired her. Those honest thoughts and feelings of fears for herself and her children will, however, remain locked within her.

Giving Advice

Another common error is to give advice to a client under the guise of helping. Giving advice means solving problems or making decisions for the client. It implies "that you know what is best and that the person is incapable of self-direction" (Murray & Zentner, 1985, p. 103).

Giving advice prevents the client from becoming independent. It prolongs the client's dependency upon the helping situation and relationship. As long as the client likes the advice and the advice given solves his or her problems, the client will continue to engage in the relationship. This relationship, however, is not a helping one because it does not encourage growth. It prohibits the client from making decisions and acting independently. It encapsulates the client, giving a false sense of security. For the day may come when the advice is not good—when the helper is blamed because things did not work out. In real life, guardian angels are nonexistent, and helpers should never attempt to assume this role. The role of advice giver can, for a time, be comforting to both client and helper. The client is relieved of the responsibility to make decisions—to be accountable in the situation. The helper can assume a role of superiority in which he or she knows all the answers to all the problems. To the client, the helper becomes all-knowing—the person with all the answers. We all know there are no perfect beings, however. We are human, and making decisions for ourselves, realistically, is a big enough task. As helpers, we cannot and must not solve other people's problems. Consider the following situation:

> About two weeks ago, Ann asked Mary for some advice about how to accomplish homework assignments better. Ann felt that Mary really knew what she was doing in school because her work was always completed and she had excellent grades. Mary was flattered by Ann's interest and quickly devised a study plan and organized a homework schedule for Ann. It is now two weeks later, and Ann finds that

the plan is not working. Her grades are dropping, and she feels inadequately prepared for classroom discussion.

Ann:	That study plan you designed for me is not working.
Mary:	It works for me—I always get everything done.
Ann:	Yeah—I know that, but you and I are two different people. I'm not you!
Mary:	Maybe you should give it more of a chance—a little more time.
Ann:	If I give it more time, I may flunk out. I was doing better on my own.

When Ann comments to Mary that they are "two different people," she has clearly summed up the major hazard of giving advice. We can only truly know ourselves. We do not have the right to solve problems for people who are capable. To do so creates an unhealthy situation, producing a dependent client.

Beginning helpers are often guilty of advising people because they think this is an effective way of helping. Clients are often willing to return for more advice—as long as things seem to be going well. Mary tries to give Ann more advice by telling her to wait—to give the study plan more time. However, Ann recognizes that the advice has not helped her, and she is now ready to think things through and solve her own problems. Helpers must be honest with clients and inform them that the purpose of the helping relationship is not to solve the problem. The function of the relationship is to help the client become an individual who is independent and accountable for his or her own actions.

Probing

Although asking questions is often necessary, in the therapeutic interaction, asking too many questions can be detrimental to the process. As stated in the previous chapter, repeated questioning of a client closes the door to the therapeutic process. Many authorities in communication skills refer to this non-therapeutic technique as *probing*. Probing is a technique in which the helper asks the client many questions without any regard for how the client is feeling about the questions. This whole area of asking questions of clients is one that presents a lot of difficulty to most helpers. We are faced with a dilemma. Should we or should we not ask the client questions? If we do not ask questions, sometimes we cannot get the necessary information to assist in our understanding of the client and the problem. To be sure, there is a "fine line" to be drawn here—questioning can be and is a necessary technique, helpful in data collection. The "fine line," however, occurs when the questioning becomes probing. Note the following example:

Rhonda is talking to her high school guidance counselor. Mr. D'accola, about her home situation.

Rhonda:	My mom died about two years ago, and my dad remarried six months ago.
Counselor:	Oh, what did your mother die of?
Rhonda:	She had cancer of the bone. She was sick for a long time.
Counselor:	And your dad just remarried?
Rhonda:	Yeah, and my stepmother is really a pain.
Counselor:	How old is your stepmother?
Rhonda:	Thirty-eight—I think.
Counselor:	How does your dad relate to you?

In this instance, the counselor's questions lack direction, serve no useful purpose, and are not helping the client. The counselor has not once responded to Rhonda's feelings. He has not tried to encourage Rhonda to focus in on one problem. Instead, the counselor seems to be introducing several new topics by asking how her mother died, about her father's remarriage, and about her relationship with her father. The question regarding Rhonda's stepmother's age seems entirely inappropriate and out of context. Questions such as the one about age are often asked out of curiosity with no real purpose intended.

Questions can make the client feel defensive, uncomfortable, confused, or threatened. The client may not know the answer to the counselor's question. Note the following example:

Amy enters Beth's room and finds her crying.

Amy:	Why are you crying?
Beth:	I don't know.
Amy:	What's the matter?
Beth:	I'm depressed. I don't know what's happening.
Amy:	There must be something going on—why are you depressed?
Beth:	I just don't know! [*Appears very irritable and hostile to Amy*]

All of us ask why once in a while—and occasionally we do get an answer and the process continues. In this instance, Amy is abusing the "why" type of question. She keeps asking Beth the same things over and over without hearing Beth's response. Beth is feeling pressured—how can she answer the question? She truly does not know why she is depressed; she only knows that she is feeling depressed. Beth is becoming irritated with Amy's form of questioning and demonstrates this feeling by shouting out her last, "I just don't know!"

Changing the Subject

Sometimes the helper abruptly changes the topic during the conversation. This is known as changing the subject or shifting the focus of conversation. A counselor who continually changes the topic is not considering the client's needs. Note the following example:

Renee is a 29-year-old woman in the process of seeking counseling for marital problems. She is presently trying to tell her counselor about her feelings concerning her husband's lack of financial assistance.

Renee: He's so cheap. He refuses to help pay the children's dentist bills! [*Voice tone is very angry*]

Counselor: Has everything else been OK—are you managing living on your own?

Renee: Yes, I'm fine—I'm just furious with him—he can well afford to help me financially.

Counselor: Where did your husband find an apartment? Near you?

In this example, the counselor has not focused on the client's feelings or even attempted to listen to what she is saying. Instead the counselor tries to introduce new subjects that have nothing to do with the client's introductory statements or her anger. Sometimes helpers abruptly change topics because they are uncomfortable with discussing the client's problems and by changing the subject they can avoid discussing something that may be unpleasant to them personally. Perhaps, in the example just given, the counselor was a male involved in paying alimony!

Minimizing the Client's Feelings

When the client does talk to the helper about feelings, it is important that the helper not minimize the client's feelings. To minimize feelings means to belittle how the client feels and to imply that these feelings are unimportant. All clients who ask for help do so because of their thoughts and feelings about particular problems or issues. Each client's thoughts and feelings are important—more important at that time than anyone else's in the world. Consider the following example:

Karen is a new mother; she delivered a seven-pound baby boy on Sunday. It is Tuesday morning, and the nurse finds her crying.

Nurse: Would you like to talk?

Karen: [*Sobbing*] Yes, I'm so upset—I don't know if I'll be able to cope.

Nurse: New mothers usually feel the way you do . . . you'll feel better in a couple of days.

Not only is the nurse telling Karen that her feelings are no different from anyone else's; she is also telling her that she *must* feel better in a couple of days. The nurse is not treating Karen as an individual with unique feelings. The client wants her thoughts and feelings to be recognized as important. She does not want them to be simply equated with the thoughts and feelings of everyone else. Although it can be somewhat comforting to know that she is not the only patient who feels this way, it is important that this client know that her "usual" feelings are being regarded by a concerned helper as "special."

Trite Expressions

Trite expressions may be used in conjunction with minimizing statements. It is easy to develop the habit of blocking effective communication by combining techniques that act as barriers. Trite expressions are glib remarks that do not encourage the client to discuss feelings and do not assist the helper to explore the client's feelings. Trite expressions often are verbalized spontaneously with no forethought as to the outcome of the communication process. Consider the following example:

> *Tom:*   I flunked the Algebra exam!
>
> *Teacher:* You flunked?
>
> *Tom:*   I didn't see the last two pages—I didn't answer 25 percent of the questions.
>
> *Teacher:* Well, it's over and done with. You can't cry over spilled milk. Let's wait and see how you do.

The teacher's final remark is in no way helpful. It merely tells Tom to stop acting upset, completely ignoring Tom's feelings. Trite remarks close the door to the communication process. In this example, Tom is being told to forget about his feelings. The teacher's statement is so final that Tom has no other recourse but to keep quiet about flunking the exam (with the teacher, anyway). Tom leaves this situation without fully expressing himself.

Jumping to Conclusions

Sometimes the helper jumps to conclusions before carefully evaluating the client's situation. The helper actually encourages the client to make a premature decision in a situation where there are usually not sufficient data to make this decision (Duldt, Giffin, & Patton, 1984). The helper is guilty of responding too quickly without really listening to all that the client has to say. The helper does not attempt to explore with the client many possible solutions. Instead, the helper encourages the client to choose the first appropriate option, which may not be the best solution. Consider the following example:

> Liz and Sally are shopping. Liz is in a hurry because she has a lot to do when she gets home. Sally has $75 to spend on an outfit for homecoming. She has just found a $65 dress for homecoming and is considering buying it.
>
> *Liz:*   That dress looks fine.
>
> *Sally:* I really like it, but I thought I'd get more wear out of a skirt and sweater.
>
> *Liz:*   But this looks nice. Why be so practical?
>
> *Sally:* [*Reluctantly*] Yeah, I guess you are right.
>
> After purchasing the dress, Sally goes home and thinks about her purchase. While reflecting upon the situation, she decides that she should have looked in the local discount stores and is upset that she only considered this one option.

In this situation Liz wanted to get home—she really did not want to investigate with Sally any of the other alternatives available. As a helper Liz is being overly assertive and dominating—she is not encouraging Sally to think the situation out and to explore all the options. In effect, Liz is solving the problem for Sally. As stated earlier, it is not within the helper's prerogative to solve the client's problems—a mistake the new helper often makes. In fact, if the client is unable to leave with a solution, the helper feels that the lesson has been a failure. This reasoning is not appropriate for helping situations. Certainly, problem solving is a desired eventual outcome in the helping situation, but to try to solve a problem prematurely severely limits the scope of the relationship and the effectiveness of the helper.

Inappropriate Use of Facts

Occasionally, helpers who have specific knowledge (i.e., nurses) use factual information inappropriately. Inappropriate use of facts means to relay information to a client that is not pertinent to that particular moment in time. The client may be so emotionally upset about a particular problem that the processing of factual material is out of the question. Sometimes helpers become overly concerned with giving factual information; they forget that their first responsibility is to help the client get "in touch" with feelings. Consider the following example:

Claire is an unwed college student who finds herself 2 months pregnant. She has made an appointment at an abortion clinic and is discussing the details with a nurse.

Claire: I'm about 2 months along . . . it's hard to believe a real person is alive inside me.

Nurse: Well, at 2 months the procedure is simple; you won't be in any danger.

Claire: I have to be here Monday at 7 A.M.—I just don't know.

Nurse: Monday at 7 A.M. will be fine. You'll have some medication and it will be all over by noon. You can leave at 1 P.M.

Claire: I've really got to think about this a lot before Monday.

In this situation the nurse seems to be "directly opposing or ignoring the views or feelings of the patient" (Hewitt & Pesznecker, 1964, p. 103). Even though Claire is giving many obvious clues that she would like to discuss her feelings, the nurse's only concern seems to be that of giving Claire the factual information related to the abortion procedure. Although the purpose of this factual information is to acquaint the client with the procedures at the abortion clinic, the nurse is not using this knowledge in an appropriate manner. The nurse has not once responded to the patient's cues, nor has the nurse considered the patient's readiness for learning. "This mode of interaction tends to weaken the relationship between nurse and patient" (Hewitt & Pesznecker, 1964, p. 103). In creating a more therapeutic interaction, the nurse must first allow the patient to express her feelings about the abortion. The technique of just giving facts demonstrates to the patient that her feelings are unimportant—that she is viewed as just another pregnant patient.

Interruption

Another error that the helper may make is to interrupt, before the client has had a chance to discuss feelings. Interruption occurs when the helper continually causes a break in the flow of the conversation by verbally interjecting remarks that prevent the client from completing the presentation of his or her ideas. There are times when it is appropriate to interrupt, especially when the client's statements seem to wander. This type of interruption is facilitative because its purpose it to help the client focus on one issue. However, there are many instances in which interruption is detrimental to the communication process. Interrupting remarks "cut the client off"—prevent a client from fully expressing his or her ideas. Note the following example:

> Frank is feeling very anxious about his impending engagement to Janet. He is having a lot of second thoughts and is not sure that he wants to get married. He is trying to talk to Mike, his best friend, about some of his doubts.
>
> *Mike:*   Well, you're a free man until Christmas—once she gets the ring you're a marked man! [*Laughing*]
> *Frank:*   Yeah. [*Looking down*]
> *Mike:*   Hey, I'm only kidding. Janet is dynamite.
> *Frank:*   You know Mike—she is far from . . .
> *Mike:*   Hey man, I'm really jealous.
> *Frank:*   She's really not as . . .
> *Mike:*   Yeah, lots of guys are envious of you; she is a super-looking lady.
> *Frank:*   Looks aren't everything . . .
> *Mike:*   Hey, there's Ron. I gotta catch him. Talk to you later . . .

It is evident from this example that Mike's continual interruption made it impossible for Frank to verbalize his feelings. Mike interrupts constantly before Frank has a chance to complete his sentences. Apparently, Mike does not hear or see any of the cues Frank is giving him.

Many of us are not aware of how we communicate, and we interrupt without ever realizing that we are doing so. In this example, Mike is probably hearing Frank's introductory comments only. He seems more concerned with discussing his thoughts about Janet than listening to Frank. Thus, if we can develop better listening habits, we will be less likely to interrupt our clients.

Prolonged Silence

In conclusion, it is important to consider prolonged silence and its effect on the communication process. Prolonged silence refers to a therapeutic situation in which silence extends beyond the point of usefulness. If there are prolonged silences in the conversation, thoughts are apt to drift, and the essence of the interaction can easily be lost. Therefore, there is a nontherapeutic component to silence as well as a therapeutic component. Helpers often are uncomfortable with silence and may tend to avoid simple helping skills such as looking at the client. The client, too, begins to feel uncomfortable, and the usefulness of silence as a technique is barely apparent. This prolonged silence allows the client and the helper to ponder upon the technique—namely silence—rather than the discussion at hand.

BECOMING A SKILLED HELPER

Effective use of communication skills is important in the helping process. Therapeutic communication techniques are necessary because they help the client to focus in on thoughts and feelings, as well as to explore possible solutions to problems (Chap. 8). Often, after an introduction to nontherapeutic responses, students feel overwhelmed as they become aware of their frequent use of these responses. It is imperative that the reader remember that *all* of us are guilty from time to time of using these types of responses. The important issue is that you begin to examine more closely how you communicate with others and that you begin to think about your responses in advance. In time, you will note that you automatically avoid such things as falsely reassuring a client or using trite expressions. You will note that your concern is with the client and the client's feelings. You will find that you are comfortable focusing on the client's problem. When you arrive at this point, you have become a helper—a facilitator!

IMPORTANT REMINDERS

1. Barriers to communication are obstacles that prevent or block the therapeutic communication process.
2. Nontherapeutic responses, also, act as barriers to effective communication.
3. Falsely reassuring a client minimizes the importance of unique feelings and promises the client a positive outcome that cannot always be guaranteed.
4. Giving advice encourages the client's dependency upon the helper and prevents the client from making his or her own decisions.
5. Probing is inappropriate questioning that makes the client feel defensive.
6. Changing the subject shifts the client's focus, thus preventing the client from carefully investigating one problem at a time.
7. When the client's feelings are minimized, the helper fails to recognize the client's need for being regarded as a unique individual.

8. Trite expressions are remarks that close the door to the communication process and prevent the client from expressing true feelings.
9. Helpers who jump to conclusions about the client's problems prevent the client from exploring all available options.
10. The helper who utilizes facts inappropriately does not consider the client's particular needs and feelings at that given moment in time.
11. A helper who continually interrupts disregards the client's need to express feelings and ideas.
12. Prolonged silences often make both client and helper uncomfortable, thus allowing both to lose the focus of the discussion.

REFERENCES

Duldt, B. W., Giffin, K., & Patton, B. R. (1984). *Interpersonal communication in nursing.* Philadelphia: Davis.

Hewitt, J., & Pesznecker, B. (1964). Blocks to communicating with patients. *American Journal of Nursing, 64,* 101–103.

Murray, B. J., & Zentner, J. P. (1985). *Nursing concepts for health promotion* (2nd ed.). Englewood Cliffs, NJ: Prentice-Hall.

Parry, J. (1968). *The psychology of human communication.* New York: American Elsevier.

Sundeen, S. J., Stuart, G. W., Rankin, E. D., & Cohen, S. A. (1985). *Nurse-client interaction implementing the nursing process.* St. Louis: C. V. Mosby.

Those who would make us feel—must feel themselves.

Charles Churchill, The Rosciad

8

Therapeutic Communication

Upon completion of the following reading and the suggested activities, the student will be able to:

1. Name and describe the following therapeutic communication skills:
   Broad opening statement
   Reflection
   Verbalization of the implied
   Seeking clarification
   Silence
   Placing events in a time sequence
   Offering oneself
   Summarization.
2. Identify the effect of these skills upon the communication process.
3. Analyze the effects of these skills upon the communication process.
4. Practice using therapeutic communication skills in role-playing situations.
5. Analyze and evaluate his or her own use of therapeutic communication skills.
6. Write a process recording.

7. Analyze and evaluate his or her own use of therapeutic and nontherapeutic communication skills.
8. Define interviewing.
9. Describe the three phases of interviewing—introductory, managing and termination.

PURPOSE OF COMMUNICATION SKILLS

Most people who enter the helping professions often find that they have a need to develop special language skills if they are to be facilitative in their relationships with clients. It is not unusual for beginning helpers to say that they did not know how to respond to the client or that they did not know what to say next. The practice of relying on previously learned social skills used strictly for developing friendships has proved to be unsuccessful when attempting to establish a therapeutic relationship with a client. Therefore, helping professionals have developed special language skills, called therapeutic communication techniques, which aid in developing more effective relationships with clients. "Therapeutic communication permits and encourages a mutuality or sharing throughout the nurse–client relationship" (Sundeen, Stuart, Rankin, & Cohen, 1985, p. 113). If used correctly, therapeutic skills help the client to verbalize feelings, to identify and assess problem areas, and to evaluate actions.

When first learning the skills of therapeutic communication, the beginning helper may feel a sense of artificiality. The skills are merely techniques at this point—they have not become part of the helper's professional personality. The beginner must learn to develop a personal style of communicating therapeutically. If used conscientiously, these skills are tools that will assist the helper in developing a therapeutic rapport with clients. The intent of this chapter is not to give hard and fast rules regarding communication skills, but to teach the beginning helper some effective methods of communicating. It is suggested that the reader slowly and consistently develop skill in using these new techniques and gradually incorporate them into patterns of communicating with clients.

There is no right or wrong method of helping someone with a problem. In fact, styles of helping are very individual, and each of us develops our own unique style. Techniques that are very effective for one person may be utterly useless for another. Helpers who are truly successful with clients need to know more than the proper communication techniques. These helpers must develop a way of demonstrating to the client that they care about the client as a person, or expert use of therapeutic communication skills is totally ineffectual.

Even when these skills are used by an experienced helper, it must be remembered that the final outcome of a therapeutic interaction does not necessarily make the client feel better! The purposes of a therapeutic interaction are to help the client to clarify and to ventilate thoughts and feelings, and to take action to change the present situation if the client believes this is necessary. The beginning helper's goal should primarily be to help the client identify and verbalize thoughts and feelings. Certainly, helping the client to solve a problem is important, but it is *not* the first task. A word of caution—remember to let a client solve his or her own problems! Decisions made by the helper for the client may later present problems for the continuation of an effective helping relationship.

As stated previously, professional helpers have developed therapeutic communication techniques to assist in establishing effective relationships with clients. The purpose of this chapter is to discuss the importance of using these skills, as well as to indicate how to use them appropriately. The therapeutic techniques discussed in this chapter are broad opening statements, reflection, verbalization of the implied, seeking clarification, silence, placing the event in time or sequence, offering one's self, and summarization. (This is by no means a final list of the techniques that could be used.) Although many of the techniques are very helpful, there are, generally, drawbacks to most techniques if they are overused or used inappropriately. Therefore, another purpose of this chapter is to help the beginner identify the strengths and weaknesses of specific therapeutic communication skills, thereby facilitating more realistic and effective use of techniques.

SOME THERAPEUTIC TECHNIQUES

Broad Opening Statements

The use of broad opening statements can be very effective when entering into a therapeutic conversation. They assist in encouraging the client "to take initiative in introducing topics and to think through problems" (Murrary & Zentner, 1985, p. 95). Statements such as, "Let's talk," or "Tell me more about yesterday," are examples of lead phrases or beginning statements. Broad opening statements allow the client an opportunity to begin focusing on feelings and defining problems. If used correctly, broad opening statements avoid the pitfalls of close-ended statements—namely, they avoid directing the client. They encourage the client to establish priorities for discussion.

Although the intent of broad opening statements is to initiate conversation, this technique is often used incorrectly. Rather than using statements such as "Let's talk about it" or "Being in the hospital can be frightening," the helper often asks specific questions such as "Why are you afraid?" Questions that ask "why" tend to make the client feel uncomfortable and defensive, as often the client is unable to answer the question. This creates a stressful rather than helpful situation.

Certainly there are occasions when it is necessary to ask questions to gather pertinent information. However, if too many direct questions are asked, the client may decrease verbalization of significant feelings and thoughts. Although the client may seemingly answer all of the helper's questions, the client's input into the relationship may be minimal. The relationship will be a superficial one of little therapeutic value to the client.

A look at the following two examples will help to clarify some of the above comments:

> You enter a hospital room and find Mrs. Jones, aged 50, crying. This is Mrs. Jones' third postoperative day after the removal of her right breast. You have taken care of her on two previous occasions. Which one of the following statements would be appropriate to begin your conversation with Mrs. Jones?
>
> 1. "Mrs. Jones, why are you crying?"
> 2. "Mrs. Jones, you really seem upset—would you like to talk?"
> 3. "Now, Mrs. Jones, you're worrying about your surgery again, aren't you?"

The first response is very limiting and puts Mrs. Jones on the spot. She may, in fact, not know why she is crying. She may also not want to discuss the fact that she is crying with the nurse. Focusing on her behavior (crying) may make her feel uncomfortable or embarrassed.

The third response is making an assumption without first accurately assessing the situation. The question asked of the patient is very "closed-ended," allowing the patient to answer with a "yes" or "no" response and, perhaps, preventing her from discussing her concerns with you.

The second question is the more appropriate of the three because it allows the patient the freedom to talk but it does not place the patient in a defensive position, nor does the nurse assume to know what is the matter.

> Your college roommate has just learned that he has failed three out of five courses he took this semester. You find him sitting at his desk staring blankly at his books. You were not aware of his difficulties in school. The conversation begins:
>
> A. *You:*   Boy, you look down!
>   *Roommate:*   Well, I guess you won't be seeing me around here anymore.
>   *You:*   I won't? Want to talk about it?
>   *Roommate:*   I'm quitting school, or rather I'm flunking out.
>   *You:*   Oh?
>   *Roommate:*   Yeah—my folks are going to be mad after spending all that money.
>   *You:*   You seem worried about your parents' reaction.
>
> B. *Roommate:*   Well, I guess you won't be seeing me around here anymore.
>   *You:*   What do you mean—I won't be seeing you?
>   *Roommate:*   I'm quitting school, or rather I'm flunking out.

You: You're kidding—that can't be true!
Roommate: I'm not joking.
You: I don't believe it!

In comparing example A with example B, it is easy to see that the first example encourages the client to focus on the problem and his feelings concerning the problem. A simple statement such as, "Oh?" from the helper encouraged the client to talk. Also, the helper continued to encourage the client when he asked, "Want to talk about it?" This statement shows that he has some feelings for the client and that he cares about him. In example B, the helper reacted emotionally and kept making the client repeat his initial statement about failing school. Without the use of a broad opening statement or other open-ended comments, this conversation seems nontherapeutic. It is almost as if the client is assuming the helping role as he tries to make the helper understand what has happened.

Reflection

"Reflecting is directing back to the client his ideas, feelings, questions, or content" (Sundeen et al., 1985, p. 116). Reflection is a technique in which the helper either repeats or restates what the client has stated for the purpose of helping the client clarify thoughts. Carl Rogers (1957) states that the aim of reflection is to understand the attitudes of the client by entering the client's internal frame of reference. The main purpose of reflection is to enable the client "to see his own attitudes, confusions, ambivalences, and perceptions accurately . . . expressed by another person . . . , but with a new quality stripped of the complications of emotion" (Carkhuff & Berenson, 1977, p. 62). The use of this technique helps the client to view problems more clearly. It gives a more objective picture of the situation, since the helper has either repeated or restated the client's stated thoughts or feelings, omitting the emotional overtones. The helper does not impose or interject any new ideas for the client to consider.

Beginning helpers have little difficulty incorporating reflection into their repertoire of therapeutic skills. To the unskilled beginner, reflection involves listening to a few key words and phrases and repeating them back to the client. In helping situations, reflection has often become an overused and overemphasized technique demonstrating the limited ability of the helper to be effective in a therapeutic sense.

Although beginners may rely heavily upon this technique, they usually complain that they feel a sense of "phonyness" when engaging in reflection. Apparently, reflection is one technique that can be used without much internalizing by the user. The beginner may be keenly aware of the fact that reflection is being used, may develop a sense of uneasiness about merely restating key phrases the client has used, and may even sense that the ability to concentrate fully on what the client is saying is lost. Thus, communication is limited because the helper focuses on merely repeating what the client is saying, rather than listening to what the client is saying. Obviously, repeated use of reflection as the only technique of therapeutic communication is a limited, stilted approach. To some, the technique is so simple to learn that the effect is never given consideration. As with the use of any technique, the helper must decide whether or not the skill is encouraging the client to clarify thoughts and to focus in on problems. It is this outcome (or the effect of the skill in encouraging the patient to communicate) that is important, not the degree of competence the helper develops when using the skill. Consider the following example:

> *Patient:* I'm so discouraged, I thought I'd be home from the hospital today.
> *Doctor:* You're discouraged?
> *Patient:* Yes, I thought I'd feel fine after surgery.
> *Doctor:* You thought you'd bounce right back to normal.
> *Patient:* Yes, in the past I've always felt great by my third postoperative day.

In this example, the doctor is using reflection as an attempt to focus in on the patient's feelings. The doctor first merely attempts to restate what the patient had said. Note that the doctor emphasized the patient's feelings of being discouraged. In the second response, the doctor rewords what the patient said, again placing emphasis upon the patient's feelings. In this example, reflection was utilized in an effective fashion. The doctor was able to identify key phrases and thoughts of the patient and was able to reflect these to the patient with relative ease, thereby encouraging further communication.

The following is another example of how reflection can be a helpful technique:

> *Linda:* I can't go to the senior dance with Joe.
> *Sue:* Oh . . . ?
> *Linda:* My parents won't let me go with him.
> *Sue:* Your parents won't let you go!
> *Linda:* No. If they find out I've been dating him, they will ground me.
> *Sue:* Find out?
> *Linda:* Yeah, I've been seeing him without my parents' permission.

In this example of reflection, Sue reports verbatim one of Linda's statements. In doing so, Sue helps to keep the conversation flowing and helps Linda to remain on the topic of discussing Joe. Sue's first comment merely indicates to Linda that she is listening and interested. Sue's third response, however, is more selective. She decided to repeat the key phrase of "find out" rather than "ground you." Since she has chosen the former key words to focus on, Linda will be able to discuss her feelings about dating Joe without her parents' knowledge. If Sue had chosen to focus her attention on the words "ground me," the discussion may not have reached the same depth. It is quite likely that Linda would have reacted to the punishment rather than her feelings. Selectivity of key words and phrases stated by the client can be an extremely important factor when engaging in therapeutic interactions. Clients often repeat the same words or phrases on several different occasions during the course of a conversation, thus making the helper's job of deciding which phrase to select easier.

Rodney Smith, patient:	I have pain in my shoulder.
Nancy Dunn, physical therapist:	You have pain?
Rodney:	Yes, severe pain in my right shoulder. It really hurts.
Nancy:	Your right shoulder is really painful.
Rodney:	I've told you twice my right shoulder hurts; can't you do something?

It is obvious in this example that the physical therapist is doing nothing more than repeating key phrases. Finally, the patient becomes exasperated with the mere parroting of his comments. In this situation, the therapist should have been more assertive in her approach, and should have attempted to elicit additional information concerning the location and the type of pain the patient was experiencing. The patient was asking for some relief. His thoughts and feelings did not need to be clarified. Thus, reflection was used inappropriately. The patient knew he was having pain and needed something more than a mere elaboration of that fact. "Too frequent and indiscriminate use of reflection might convey to the patient . . . distinterest and inattentiveness. Parroting and mimicry can make nondirective techniques ludicrous and block communication" (Collins, 1977, p. 79). In emphasizing the latter points, consider the following:

Al Capone, prisoner:	This place is awful! I've got to get out!
Bob Litch, counselor:	The jail is awful?
Prisoner:	You know what the food is like, and you've seen our cells.
Counselor:	You feel it's awful?
Prisoner:	Well, what do you think?

In this example, the counselor began immediately to use reflection. He only focused on the first half of the prisoner's opening comment, perhaps entirely missing the prisoner's purpose in bringing up this topic for conversation. Although this prisoner will probably never discuss "getting out" with this counselor, it is very likely that this is what he had in mind when he began the conversation. The counselor's responses, although reflective, may not have been the most appropriate at this time. His further comments do not capture any feelings for the client, but rather they seem to evoke anger as the client very curtly asks the counselor, "What do you think?"

Verbalization of the Implied

Reflection is often used with another similar technique called verbalization of the implied. When using verbalization of the implied, the helper does more than restate or reword what the client has already said. The helper instead adds to what the client states, thus encouraging the client to continue with the conversation and to focus on the problem. The following example illustrates how verbalization of the implied differs from reflection:

> *Lisa Howe, patient:*   I'm so discouraged. I thought I'd be home from the hospital today.
>
> *Joan Lathin, nurse:*   You're discouraged because you're still in the hospital.
>
> *Patient:*   Yes, I thought I'd feel fine after surgery.
>
> *Nurse:*   The surgery took more out of you than you anticipated.
>
> *Patient:*   Yes. In the past after surgery, I've always looked forward to returning home and resuming my household responsibilities, but this time . . .
>
> *Nurse:*   This time you're dreading it.
>
> *Patient:*   I just don't think I can do it—the kids require so much attention—I'm really afraid I'll be sick again.

As you can see from this example, the nurse has encouraged the patient to discuss her feelings and her problem. Rather than repeating to the patient similar phrases that she has already used, the nurse responds by adding to what the patient has said. This type of technique often helps the patient to clearly identify concerns. Both techniques can be helpful tools when interacting with clients. Reflection is very helpful when you really have no ideas about what is worrying the client. Verbalization of the implied becomes more useful once you have developed a rapport with your client and you have more insight into the client's thoughts and feelings.

Seeking Clarification

Seeking clarification is extremely important in a therapeutic relationship and should be accomplished as soon as the helper recognizes there is confusion about what the client is saying. Seeking clarification is an attempt by the helper to understand the client's situation clearly by asking the client to clarify certain information that is vague or not meaningful. It is often difficult to admit confusion or lack of understanding and, therefore, the helper may allow the client to continue to discuss irrelevant information. In allowing this to happen, the helper is wasting time that is very precious to the client and overlooking the fact that a serious problem may be underlying the client's vague conversation.

It is not unusual for the client involved in a stressful situation to be somewhat confused about his or her thoughts and feelings. Sometimes, when attempting to communicate therapeutically with such a client, the helper will note that the client tends to ramble from one topic to another, having a great deal of difficulty defining problems. The following example illustrates the previous point:

Patient:	I never expected to have a G.I. series today.
Nurse:	Oh?
Patient:	I'm really angry with my husband about last night.
Nurse:	You're mad at your husband?
Patient:	I wonder how long I'll have to stay in the hospital.

Although the nurse is attempting to use therapeutic skills to encourage the patient to talk, the results of the nurse's efforts are disappointing. Rather than responding to the nurse's leads (such as "Oh?" or "You're really mad at your husband?") the patient continues to ramble.

If the nurse does not intervene at an appropriate time, the entire conversation may continue in this fashion. If the nurse does not help the patient to clarify her thoughts, this communication encounter will be fruitless. The patient will be left in a state of confusion. Furthermore, the patient may begin to develop doubts about the nurse, who seemed to listen to her but did not have any input into the interaction. Patients are perceptive and recognize early those who pretend to understand but do not. There is nothing wrong with simply saying to the patient, "I'm sorry; I'm confused about the point you are trying to make." If this is done in an unobstrusive fashion, demonstrating a true interest for the patient and what she is saying, the patient may try to reorganize her thoughts and to present them in a clearer manner. Thus, by approaching the situation honestly, the patient has been given the chance to clarify vague statements and to try to place her thoughts into proper perspective.

> It is not necessary to understand everything he says as long as you are honest about it and do not pretend to understand what you do not. Attempting to discover what the person is talking about can help him become clearer to himself. (Murray & Zentner, 1985, p. 97)

The second example illustrates another situation where the helper asks for clarification inappropriately.

Jarrod Long, student:	I'm dropping my advanced math course this semester.
Mr. Harris, counselor:	Do you think that's a wise decision?
Jarrod Long:	Yes. I'm getting a D in the course, and I feel that will bring my 3.5 cumulative average down.
Mr. Harris:	But I don't understand—you need the course to graduate.
Jarrod Long:	Yes, I need to pass the course to graduate, and I feel I will do better taking it next semester.

Mr. Harris:	Why not try to pass the course this semester? If you fail it, you can always take it again next semester.
Jarrod Long:	Because a failure will hurt my cumulative average.

This student is presenting his thoughts and feelings quite clearly to the counselor. The counselor, however, does not seem to hear what the student is saying and tells him rather inappropriately that he needs the course for graduation. The counselor seems to ignore the client's feelings about receiving a failing grade. It would be understandable if this client reacted with distrust toward this counselor. The student may decide that this particular counselor does not listen when he tries to share a problem with him and will, therefore, decide to close the door to becoming involved with this counselor. The counselor did not listen to what the student was saying. Therefore, since he did not give the client his full attention, he demonstrated a lack of interest in the client and his problem.

Silence

Silence is a communication technique that allows the helper and client to interact without the use of words. This nonverbal method of communicating can be very effective if used appropriately. Silence provides the client with an opportunity to collect and organize his or her thoughts without interruption. Used correctly, it relays the message that talking is not a necessary criterion for the relationship. If the silence is a positive one, the client gains a feeling of self-worth and self-respect. The client views the helper as a person who is concerned and who is willing to wait for the client to give the cues as to when and if the conversation will begin again.

Although silence is one of the more effective therapeutic skills, it requires a person of competence to employ it correctly. Socially, most of us simply do not feel comfortable with silences; if there are lulls in the conversation, we feel something is wrong. Therefore, it is not unusual to have the helper enter into this kind of relationship with the same feelings. "Helpers often feel compelled to break silences because of their own feelings of self-consciousness and embarrassment" (Collins, 1977, p. 90). The helper needs to practice this skill frequently before mastering it. Silence allows both the helper and client "a golden opportunity to contemplate thoughtfully what has been said and felt, to weigh alternatives, to formulate new ideas, and to gain a new perspective of the matter under discussion" (Collins, 1977, p. 70). The following examples are given to illustrate how silence as a technique can be utilized:

Dorothy is a 72-year-old female who has just died somewhat unexpectedly. Her husband, Jacob, is sitting in the room holding her hand. Their rabbi, who has known the family for years, enters the room.

Rabbi: Jacob, I just want you to know that I'm here if you need anything [*puts hand on Jacob's shoulder and sits next to him*].

Jacob: Thank you. You've been so kind throughout this ordeal. [*talks quietly, looking at rabbi*]

Rabbi: I want you to know I'm really sorry.

Jacob: It was just so sudden—I can't believe she's gone. [*Sobs gently, putting head in palms of hands*]

Rabbi: [*Puts arm around Jacob's shoulders, looks directly at him, and sits quietly waiting for Jacob to give the next verbal cue.*]

In this example, the helper demonstrates his ability to utilize silence in an effective and comfortable fashion. The rabbi has told Jacob that he is available to help and that he is sorry, verbally demonstrating his concern. However, the rabbi's nonverbal, silent response further reinforces his concern. He devotes his entire attention to Jacob and allows Jacob to weep without attempting to interrupt the silence, thus allowing him ample time to collect his thoughts.

Sandy is a 14-year-old girl who has been truant from school quite frequently. The family court has assigned Sandy a counselor, Eric Savich, to whom she must report on a weekly basis. Sandy is presently meeting with her counselor. Yesterday, the truant officer found her at home rather than in school and has reported this to the counselor.

Counselor: I see you missed another day of school.

Sandy: Yeah. [*She offers no other response and stares at floor*]

Counselor: [*Becoming noticeably fidgety in his chair, breaks silence*] What happened?

Sandy: [*Offers no verbal response*]

Counselor: [*Looking at watch*] Well, Sandy, if you have nothing to say for yourself, you may as well leave.

Sandy: OK.

In this example the client is actually punished because she remains silent. The counselor dismisses Sandy because she is not talking to him. The counselor began the conversation by immediately mentioning Sandy's truant behavior. Sandy reacted rather strongly and refused to respond with any verbal information concerning the situation. "If the patient feels pressured to talk about a subject that he finds too painful, he may react with stony silence as a form of defiance or resistance" (Collins, 1977, p. 69). The counselor would have been more effective if he had not confronted Sandy immediately. Sandy may have interpreted his initial statement as a reprimand and felt that the counselor's only concern was whether she attended school or not. The counselor had some difficulty coping with Sandy's silence. He gave nonverbal cues such as fidgeting and looking at his watch during Sandy's silent periods. Verbally, he broke both silent episodes by interjecting rather punitive types of responses.

There is no rule that states a given time for which silences should last. Realistically, these periods should provide a useful function—that of allowing both client and helper an opportunity to collect their thoughts. They should not extend so long that the reason for the conversation is lost. Also, if the helper is feeling very uncomfortable and notices he or she is not able to give the client full attention, it is appropriate to interrupt silence. Interruption, however, should be done in a caring fashion where the helper responds, perhaps, to a feeling tone of the client. Reprimands such as those given by the counselor to Sandy are not appropriate and do not encourage a therapeutic interaction.

Placing the Event in Time or Sequence

Placing the event in time or sequence is a useful technique in assisting the client to develop a clearer perspective regarding a given event. When using this technique, the helper directs questions that ask for information, such as, "What happened before you felt depressed?" or "Did the pain occur before or after heavy exercise?" When asking for such information, the helper is gaining information about sequences of events and whether certain events influenced the client's response. This technique should only be used when the helper feels confident that the information obtained from the client will be used for some therapeutic purpose. Consider the following examples:

> Jim enters Bob's dormitory room looking very tense and very unhappy. It is final exam time, and the fraternity Jim wants to pledge has told him that he must steal a math exam to earn the honor of being pledged.

> *Jim:* Well, I did it.
>
> *Bob:* You did what?
>
> *Jim:* Stole the exam. Right from under poor Dr. Jones' nose. [*Eyes downcast, tone soft*]
>
> *Bob:* What happened?
>
> *Jim:* I just went into his office and took it.
>
> *Bob:* Took it while he was in the room?
>
> *Jim:* No, the poor guy trusted me in the office and left for about half an hour while I was supposedly reviewing old exams.
>
> *Bob:* So where did you find the exam?

Although Bob is doing an adequate job at placing events in a sequence and finding out exactly what occurred, he is not relating to Jim in a therapeutic fashion. Bob is more interested in what happened or, more specifically, the story of how Jim stole the exam. He ignores Jim's nonverbal cues of being tense and unhappy. Furthermore, he does not identify Jim's verbal cues of being unhappy about what he has done. Note that Jim refers to Dr. Jones as "the poor guy" twice, and he states that Dr. Jones trusted him to be in his office alone. Bob does not attempt to reflect any of Jim's feelings and, therefore, never develops a therapeutic relationship with Jim.

Joan, age 17, has always been an excellent student. In the past two months her grades have been very mediocre. Her mother has been ill for several years and Joan is responsible for caring for her two brothers, ages 8 and 10. Her teacher has asked to talk with Joan about her recent drop in grades.

Joan:	I know my grades are only fair. I should be doing better.
Teacher:	It's only been within the last two months. Has something happened at home?
Joan:	Well, you know my mom's ill and I do a lot of the work.
Teacher:	Yes—has the workload increased?
Joan:	Not really, but . . .
Teacher:	But?
Joan:	Well, about six months ago, in September, I started to work part time to save money for college.
Teacher:	But your grades were fine the first four months of school; it's only recently that they've begun to drop.
Joan:	In the last two months, I've increased my hours to almost full time because of my dad.
Teacher:	Has something happened to your father?
Joan:	Yes, he lost his job, and my family needs the money I'm making.

In this example the teacher uses a combination of reflecting, as well as placing the event in a time sequence, to help the student identify the problem. Joan has an idea that her job may be influencing her grades, but she is not really sure. The teacher astutely notes that her grades were fine six months ago and they have only begun to drop recently. By specifically stating this fact to the client, the client can better examine the time frame of events in order to identify exactly where the problem exists.

Offering Oneself

Offering oneself is one of the easier therapeutic skills to learn. Most people who enter helping professions do so because of their desire to help others. Therefore, it is reasonable to assume that most helpers will be readily available to meet with clients. Letting the client know that you have time available to talk or that you can just sit for a while has a positive influence upon any therapeutic relationship. Helpers, however, must learn to offer their help responsibly as it is virtually impossible for any one person to interact therapeutically eight hours per day. Beginning helpers must learn how to set limits with clients. Under ideal conditions, both client and helper should have an accurate perception at the outset of the approximate time available for each interaction. It is unfair and psychologically harmful to the client to be abruptly interrupted because the helper has no more time to discuss the problem.

It is ten o'clock in the morning, and Jill finds her college roommate Becky sobbing while reading a letter. Jill must be in class by 10:15, but she promises Becky that she will return immediately after class to discuss the apparent problem. Becky states that she will look forward to seeing Jill around 11:30 A.M. After class, Jill either forgets her promise or the incident because she decides to go out to lunch with a group of friends. Jill returns to the room at 3:00 P.M.

Becky: That was sure a long class. [*Rather sarcastically*]

Jill: Oh, Becky, I'm so sorry. I couldn't have gotten back earlier.

Becky: That's OK. It really wasn't that important.

Jill: I've got some time now.

Becky: I'm feeling much better—let's forget it.

Jill made a commitment to Becky, but did not keep her word. Becky receives a nonverbal message that she is not that important to Jill or Jill would have returned immediately after class. Becky's trust in Jill is disrupted, and she recognizes that she cannot depend upon Jill for help. By not returning at the agreed time (especially without notifying the client), the helper has lost her chance to be effective. Becky may interpret Jill's tardiness as reluctance on Jill's part to help with the problem. Jill has nonverbally implied that the problem is not one of real significance or she would have returned after her class to talk with Becky. Therefore, by not returning when promised, the helper has lost her chance to interact with the client therapeutically.

John is working in a fast-food restaurant. It is 11 A.M. and no customers have arrived as yet. Mark begins to talk to him about changing jobs.

John: I had no idea you wanted to leave work.

Mark: Don't tell anyone—I would like to discuss it with you before I quit.

John: Sure, I'd be glad to, but why don't we go out for a cup of coffee after work? You know what the lunch crowd does to this place at 11:30 A.M.

Mark: Great idea—see you then.

In this example, John has offered to help. By setting limits on a time to discuss Mark's decision, John has chosen the more appropriate course. He knows that he will be very busy in a few minutes and will not have time to devote totally to Mark. Even though John has chosen to delay the conversation, he has made a wise decision, since therapeutic interactions need proper external conditions such as a quiet place void of interruptions. A busy restaurant, hospital room, or classroom are certainly not ideal places to offer one's help to a client.

Summarization

All therapeutic interactions should end with a final summarization of what has taken place during the conversation. The summary will "bring together important points of discussion and give particular emphasis to progress made toward greater understanding" (Murray & Zentner, 1985, p. 98). The summary helps to close the conversation and allows both the helper and the client to reflect upon the therapeutic interaction. Consider the following example:

> Pat and Martin have been dating steadily for six months. Pat has decided that she would like to date other boys as well. She has told Martin how she feels, and he agrees that they both should date other people.
>
> Pat: I'm glad we're still friends, and I'm looking forward to continuing our relationship on a not-so-steady basis.
>
> Martin: Me too. I think we really need to spend time with other people. I'll see you in a month for the rock concert.
>
> Pat: Great . . . bye for now!

In this example, Pat ends the conversation by summarizing the important issues—namely, dating other people and continuing their present relationship on a "not-so-steady basis." Martin indicates by his closing comment that he, too, has a good understanding of what has happened during this interaction.

Summary statements need not be long and involved. Clear, concise statements indicating what has taken place are most useful to both the helper and the client. The statements afford the client an opportunity to think about what has occurred during the interaction and what course of action might be taken because of the interaction.

PROCESS RECORDING

Perhaps one of the best ways to help you to examine your ability to engage in therapeutic interactions is to have you record an actual interaction in which you attempted to help someone.

You will be asked to write a process recording at the completion of this chapter. A *process recording* is a written encounter of your interaction as a helper with a client. The most important part of this recording is your analysis of the techniques you used to help the client and the appropriateness of that technique you chose. Also, inherent in completion of this assignment is your ability to identify nonverbal as well as verbal cues of the client. Thus, writing a process recording is an assignment that helps you to recognize your strengths and weaknesses as a helper.

Unfortunately, writing down the exact interaction often presents difficulty to new helpers, since they are afraid they will not remember the entire conversation. It is not necessary to record the whole interaction; record only the part in which you attempt to intervene therapeutically. Be sure to capture the exact wording of the client immediately before and after your responses. Your written work should be done as soon after the interaction as possible.

Ideally, videotape or a tape recorder should be used for this assignment, so that the learner can see or, at least, hear him- or herself interact therapeutically. However, the use of videotape or tape recorders can make clients uncomfortable and interfere with their ability to interact. Thus, this author suggests that the beginner practice recording conversations from memory—employing the senses of seeing, touching, hearing, and smelling when making observations.

An Example

Study the process recording in Table 8–1 and critically analyze its contents. Remember, you are not expected always to respond using the correct technique. It is far more important for you to begin to recognize your weaknesses and to start to develop the skills necessary to become an effective helper.

TABLE 8-1. PROCESS RECORDING

Description of Situation:	Lisa is a 14-year-old junior high student with an apparent "father persecution" complex.		
Interaction	**Technique**	**Analysis**	**Preferred Response (When Appropriate)**
Helper: "Hi, Lisa. How are things going?"	Opening question (serves same function as broad opening statement)	Appropriate question; introduces topic.	
Lisa: "Do you really want to know?" [*tapping fingers on the table*]			
Helper: "I'm here and more than willing to listen."	Offering self	Appropriate—lets Lisa know someone will listen.	
Lisa: "I don't feel close to my dad any more."			
Helper: "Why?"	Question	"Why" response is inappropriate; reflection would be more helpful. This type of question may make a client feel defensive; Lisa may not know the answer.	"You don't feel close to your dad any more."
Lisa: "I don't really know. He always			

TABLE 8–1. PROCESS RECORDING (cont.)

Interaction	Technique	Analysis	Preferred Response (When Appropriate)
seems to be with my brothers. [*Softly*] I don't think he loves me."			
Helper: "Maybe your dad feels your mom is not giving the boys enough attention."	Changes topic	The helper did not pick up on the cue, "I don't think he loves me." Instead, the helper focuses on a reason for Lisa's father's behavior. Also, the helper noted that Lisa spoke softly about her feelings but did not recognize why she was speaking softly.	"You're really quite upset about your relationship with your dad."
Lisa: "I really thought he paid attention to me before, but since my grandfather died, he has barely spoken to me."			
Helper: "Well, that's probably the reason for his closeness to your brothers. He is trying to build a relationship with his sons and probably does not realize that he is excluding you."	Changes topic; jumps to a conclusion without knowing all the facts.	The helper is focusing on the father and his actions rather than on the client. It would have been better for the helper to seek clarification about when this change took place and how the client feels about it.	"You noticed a change at the time of your grandfather's death. How long ago was that?" (Time-sequencing)
Lisa: "I hadn't thought about it that way before."			
Helper: I know it hurts now, but	False reassurance,	Inappropriate—the helper really	"You say your father barely *(continued)*

TABLE 8-1. PROCESS RECORDING *(cont.)*

Interaction	Technique	Analysis	Preferred Response (When Appropriate)
your father really does love you. Everything will turn out OK."	trite expression.	does not know that the client's father loves her. The helper also is minimizing Lisa's feelings by never allowing her an opportunity to verbalize her feelings.	talks to you. Could you elaborate on this for me?"

After rereading this process recording, the helper recognizes that more practice in therapeutic communication skills is needed. After looking at the opening comments about describing the situation, the helper notes that a subtle but definite value judgment was made. The term "father persecution complex" is purely a biased comment made by the helper without any real information to substantiate it. Also, a statement like this indicates a diagnosis, and this is *not* the purpose of the helper in the therapeutic process. The helper also needs to pay particular attention to the focus of the conversation and attempt to direct the focus back to the client's feelings. Although glib statements and false reassurance were used, there is something in this helper's response that indicates a willingness to help. There needs, however, to be more than the innate desire to help for a communication process to be fruitful.

INTERVIEWING

While therapeutic communication techniques are commonly used in a dialogue format to elicit feelings and resolve problems, they have another application called interviewing.

Interviewing is a basic skill utilized by a variety of professionals. As defined by these authors, it is an intentional verbal interaction in which the helper guides the client in an effort to learn more about the client's situation, problems, and so on. This is frequently accomplished by asking specific questions, the content of which has been at least in part, previously determined. The art of effective interviewing is to be able to gather necessary data in a manner that is personalized and professional. The interview process can be better understood if discussed, as it occurs, in three phases of development. Figure 8–1 summarizes the important points.

Introductory Phase

The first phase is social in nature. The greetings that we have learned from childhood, such as a proper introduction and a handshake, are still essential—

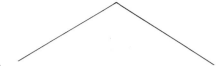

I. Introduction
Establishing social milieu; client comfort; building a rapport; exploring feelings; client cooperation; clarifying expectations

II. Management
Most time-consuming; productive, gathering information; responding to client needs; working together; continued clarification of feelings; recognition of client feelings; presentation of facts

III. Termination
Begins at first interview; helper needs to institute presummary, summary, and follow-up; appreciation of client's time and feelings important

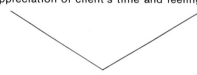

Figure 8-1. Phases of interviewing. Note that the management phase is the most expansive and productive portion. *(Adapted from Cormier et al., 1984, p. 49.)*

even more so in a professional relationship. "The ritualistic greetings . . . are important in validating the individual as a person worthy of respect and recognition" (Duldt, Giffin, & Patton, 1984, p. 247). The interviewer or the helper is responsible for conducting the interview. It is up to the helper to determine the time and place for the interview and be responsible for establishing the social milieu or mood of the interview. Have you ever felt uncomfortable during a job interview? Do you have any idea why? Client comfort and privacy is vital to the success of the entire interview. Consider the following example:

> Mrs. Daniels is a social worker at a local hospital. Her assignment for today is to begin to find nursing home placement for Mr. Harrod Jamiel, a 68-year-old retired state worker who has a diagnosis of lung cancer. Mrs. Daniels is unsure of how to proceed. She has to ask many personal questions regarding living arrangements and financial status. The nurses and the physicians have told her that Mr. Jamiel has plenty of visitors and that they appear to be quite affluent. Nurses and physicians also tell her that Mr. Jamiel has not been easy to communicate with—often he prefers not to talk.

Mrs. Daniels knows that this introductory phase is extremely important. Its purpose is to build a rapport, establish an interview schedule, and clarify expectations (Cormier, Cormier, & Weisser, 1984, p. 48).

Simple, cordial introductions are appropriate for this first task of establishing a rapport. Remember, as a professional helper, you should be using a repertoire of learned techniques that will help you to identify the verbal and nonverbal communication cues of the client. Note the following:

> *Mrs. Daniels:* Good morning, Mr. Jamiel. I'm Janice Daniels, the social worker. [*Smiles and extends her hand*]
>
> *Mr. Jamiel:* Hello. [*Looks straight ahead; does not extend hand for handshake*]
>
> *Mrs. Daniels:* I'm here to discuss nursing homes with you. We have one week to work on this project. [*Presents facts clearly and simply, describing her purpose*]
>
> *Mr. Jamiel:* So it's done; I've got to be put away in one of those awful places. [*Is direct—looks at Mrs. Daniels*]
>
> *Mrs. Daniels:* You seem angry about going.
>
> *Mr. Jamiel:* You're damn right I am!

At this point in the interview, Mrs. Daniels feels that she must focus on the client's feelings. It is clear to her that he is upset about being placed in a nursing home, and to ignore this would be counterproductive. Clarifying Mr. Jamiel's feelings and expectations would, of course, be easier if she knew something about the client and his life-style (Elder, 1978). As in any interaction of this nature, it is far more beneficial to allow the client time to explore feelings than to continue questioning and data collection.

Once the interviewer has established a rapport with the client, the interview should be structured in such a way as to be conducive to gaining necessary information. Mrs. Daniels has spent one session talking over Mr. Jamiel's feelings, and she is now ready to begin helping him choose an appropriate nursing home. She begins the session by stating:

> *Mrs. Daniels:* Well, today is the day we begin thinking about possible nursing home placement. I have about 45 minutes and several questions to ask. If you're able to answer my questions, I think I might be able to find a place suitable for your needs.

This type of statement establishes a clear agenda so the client knows what to expect.

> *Mr. Jamiel:* Shoot with the questions. If I have to go, I want to go in style. [*Laughs briefly, responds warmly. The nurses and Mr. Jamiel's family have both commented that the first meeting with Mrs. Daniels seemed to put him at ease—he really feels she is concerned about his welfare*]

During this part of the interview, Mrs. Daniels begins by asking the least threatening questions first. In the beginning she may even know some of the answers, such as where the client lives, but her intent is to make the client comfortable—to ease the client into the situation. The following is an example of the kind of interactions that take place:

> *Mrs. Daniels:* Now let me see. You live in Portland, and most of your children live near you, I think?
>
> *Mr. Jamiel:* That's right. My two sons live about a half hour away from Portland.
>
> *Mrs. Daniels:* So you'd like to go to a nursing home that is near your sons.
>
> *Mr. Jamiel:* I'd really like to be near John; he has always been more concerned about spending time with me.

Mrs. Daniels listens intently to Mr. Jamiel's answers. She knows that her ability to help is contingent upon her knowledge and understanding of his needs. Both she and Mr. Jamiel have clear expectations about what will occur as a result of this interview. There is no hidden agenda or motives. The communication is open, and both parties have a right to expect honest exchanges.

If the expectations of the interview process are clarified early in the relationship, the client will not be confused about the helper's role. Mr. Jamiel knows that Mrs. Daniels' intent is to find him placement in a nursing home. He also knows that she will do her best to find a home that suitably meets his needs. Mrs. Daniels has certain expectations, also. She expects that Mr. Jamiel will cooperate by answering questions, will be honest in his responses, and will disclose important information. If these expectations are to be met, a trusting relationship must be established.

Management Phase

The middle portion of the interview, referred to as the management phase, is the most productive and time-consuming phase (Cormier et al., 1984). In this phase, the helper is concerned with obtaining information, giving information, and responding to the client's feelings. This will help the interviewer gain a perspective about the problems that are of concern to the client. The interviewer needs to approach this phase creatively and cautiously. Questions, especially numerous questions, can hinder the helper's rapport with clients. Thus, a conscious effort should be made to gather information without always using a questioning format. Note how adept Mrs. Daniels is at doing this:

> *Mrs. Daniels:* So your son John is willing to help you out a little.
>
> *Mr. Jamiel:* Oh, yeah. He helps me pay all my accounts. He is very trustworthy.
>
> *Mrs. Daniels:* OK. Let's see what I can do about placing you in a home that is not more than 20 minutes from John. After all, we want him to continue to be able to see you. Now I need to find out a little more about your finances. I know these are personal questions,

but your answers will help me to make the proper arrangements.

Mr. Jamiel: Well, I have about $25,000 in a high-interest account and some stocks. I think I can afford to pay my way for quite a while. I thought I might not make it home last year. At that time I gave all my property to my two sons. Its worth was quite astronomical—$450,000. At least I know I've left them something.

Mrs. Daniels: That's a nice feeling. You have just one bank account? [*Making a mental note about the apparent affluence of relatives, she realizes that the client's funds may be limited for a long-term nursing home stay*]

Mr. Jamiel: Oh, I have two other small accounts with approximately $3,000 in each and about $1,000 in my checking account. [*Willingly gives information—takes out bank books to show Mrs. Daniels the three accounts*]

As you can see by this interaction, Mrs. Daniels is able to gather quite a bit of information using several techniques, not just questioning.

"As far as patients are concerned, the giving of information and instructions is the most sensitive and critical part of the interaction" (Cormier et al., 1984, p. 53). The client needs to be informed of what to expect, the options available, and the relative benefits and risks of these options. Note how Mrs. Daniels gives information to Mr. Jamiel:

Mrs. Daniels: After examining all of your financial assets and considering your personal wishes, I've decided upon two possible placements, each quite different from the other.

Mr. Jamiel: Sounds interesting—am I going to spend $25,000 in the first week?

Mrs. Daniels: No, but one option is more costly. [*Uses eye contact*]

Mr. Jamiel: Let's have the good news first. [*Smiles—intently listens to response*]

Mrs. Daniels: You could go to a halfway house—it is about 40 minutes from John's house, but the cost is half that of a nursing home.

Mr. Jamiel: Well, what's the difference? Is a nursing home better?

Mrs. Daniels: No—one is not better than the other. In the halfway house you would have to assume more of your own care. The professional nursing staff is limited.

Mr. Jamiel: So if I begin to feel really ill, I might not have as many people there to look after me.

Mrs. Daniels: Right—and it might take a few weeks to transfer you into a nursing home. Also, there is no guarantee that you would be transferred into a home near John's.

Mr. Jamiel: Do you have a place for me now near John's?

Mrs. Daniels: Yes, I do, in a nursing home about 15 minutes from him, but they will only keep it available for one day.

Mr. Jamiel: So I need to make my decision real soon. [*Eyes downcast, voice softens*]

Mrs. Daniels: I'm afraid you do. I told them we would call by 4 P.M. tomorrow. I realize that this is not easy for you.

Mrs. Daniels has assumed a supportive role in which she has clarified information and presented facts to Mr. Jamiel. She has informed Mr. Jamiel of the available options and the consequences of choosing those options. Mrs. Daniels has been attentive to Mr. Jamiel's nonverbal and verbal communication cues. Mrs. Daniels knows her client well and recognizes that a placement in the nursing home represents for him a loss of independence—both financially and physically. She also knows that Mr. Jamiel is well aware of his medical condition and the fact that he might need more nursing care in the future. She has not, however, opted to make a choice for Mr. Jamiel—she has merely presented the facts as they exist. She does indicate to Mr. Jamiel her awareness of how difficult this choice must be. It is important that helping professionals "indicate their awareness and understanding of patient feelings and emotions as they are expressed—overtly or covertly—during the interaction" (Cormier et al., 1984, p. 54).

Terminating the Interview

Inherent in the interview process is the notion of termination, whether it be termination of a particular session or termination of the entire process. Plans for termination of the process must be "built in" from the beginning. Clients have the right to know the helper's purpose and the approximate length of time available to the helper for a particular client. Mrs. Daniels tells Mr. Jamiel at their first meeting that she plans to spend 1 week finding a nursing home placement for him. Even though Mr. Jamiel may not feel this time frame is adequate, he has been given an honest response and advanced warning that the relationship will end. Helpers must be responsible about beginning the termination process with the beginning phase of the interview process.

Most helpers are aware of this responsibility and conscientiously try to institute it in their practice. However, it is sometimes more difficult to plan for the termination of each individual session. Cormier et al. (1984) suggest that helpers use the presummary, summary, and follow-up approaches in an attempt to guarantee adequate closure at each individual session.

Approximately 10 minutes before the end of Mr. Jamiel's session, Mrs. Daniels gently reminds him that they have about 10 minutes left and asks if he would like to discuss any other problems. This type of statement informs the client that the session is nearing its end and provides an opportunity for the client to share a pertinent problem that may have been overlooked. Presummary statements like this make clear to the client that termination is due to time constraints, not rejection (Cormier et al., 1984). If helpers consistently follow this approach, clients will learn to expect this as part of the normal approach to all interviews.

Summary statements clarify for the client what has transpired during the interview. Note how Mrs. Daniels summarizes for Mr. Jamiel:

> *Mrs. Daniels:* Before I leave, I want to quickly review your two options—the halfway house for about half the cost, $300 a week, versus the nursing home at $600 a week. The halfway house is 40 minutes from John, and the nursing home is 15 minutes.
>
> *Mr. Jamiel:* And if I go to the halfway house and become ill, I can be moved to the nursing home.
>
> *Mrs. Daniels:* Yes, but most likely there will not be an opening in the home near John's house—you could be placed anywhere. The next nearest home to John's is an hour's drive.
>
> *Mr. Jamiel:* I need a couple of hours to think this over and to talk to John.
>
> *Mrs. Daniels:* That's a good idea; I'll stop by in the morning for your decision.

Note that no new information has been introduced. The helper has reviewed for Mr. Jamiel his options and has encouraged him to respond to her request. Summary statements "should contain your specific instructions and encourage the patient to accept responsibility" (Froelick, Bishop, & Dworkin, 1976, p. 61).

As Mrs. Daniels prepares to leave, she extends her hand to Mr. Jamiel and says, "Thank you for being so helpful. I know this is not an easy task for you, and I really appreciate your cooperation. I'll come back tomorrow for your final decision."

The interview should not be terminated without a follow-up and an expression of appreciation from the helper (Hillman, Goodell, Grundy, McArthur, & Moller, 1981). Mrs. Daniels assures Mr. Jamiel that she will return for a follow-up to learn his final decision. Helpers must not assume that the task of making decisions and/or answering questions is easy for clients. As in other helping encounters, a word of praise from a thoughtful helper can serve as an earned reward to the client.

DEVELOPING ONE'S OWN COMMUNICATION STYLE

Clearly, there is an art to therapeutic communication. One must be highly skilled in the use of therapeutic techniques and the process of interviewing. Both are learned skills that require practice and refinement. "No single approach, style or technique of interviewing is adequate" (Gorden, 1980). The helper must learn, however, to go beyond the skills used in everyday conversation to use a variety of skills appropriate for therapeutic interactions. These skills are more likely to help the client answer questions and provide much needed information to the helper. Knowledge of the skills is only part of the answer in developing effective relationships with clients. The sincere interest of the helper as a person who truly has developed positive regard for the client is far more important than the use of communication skills. Ultimately, each of you will develop your own style of helping. At first, you may feel apprehensive. It is sometimes difficult to focus on what you are saying as well as how you are saying it. Discussing information that is of a personal nature can be embarrassing. As a beginning helper, you may find using one or two techniques that seem to "fit" more practical than attempting to use all of the techniques discussed in this chapter. When these techniques have been practiced and perfected, others can be tried. Gradually, your approach to helping will become more sophisticated, and the styles used may change. This is fine, because style change, in this case, indicates growth.

The beginner needs to practice these skills frequently if mastery is to occur. Most students find that the techniques are helpful when discussing problems with friends. The client group need not come from a select population; students are encouraged to utilize these techniques whenever the opportunity presents itself.

IMPORTANT REMINDERS

1. Therapeutic communication involves skills that assist the helper in being more facilitative during the communication process.
2. Broad opening statements are lead phrases that encourage the client to direct the discussion of the problem.
3. Reflection refers to a skill in which the helper either rephrases or repeats what the client has already stated for the purpose of helping the client clarify his or her thoughts.
4. Verbalizing the implied thoughts and feelings of the client helps him or her to become more fully aware of feelings.
5. It is imperative that helpers who do not fully understand the client's feelings encourage the client to further clarify thoughts and ideas.
6. If both the helper and client are comfortable with silence, this technique can be very useful in allowing the client time to ponder his or her thoughts.
7. In some situations, it is useful for the helper to be aware of the time frame in which certain events occurred.
8. It is important that the client be aware of the helper's readiness and availability to help.
9. Summary statements afford both client and helper an opportunity to reflect upon what has taken place during the interaction.
10. Positive regard for the client is the most essential component in creating a therapeutic environment.
11. Interviewing is an intentional verbal interaction in which the helper guides the client in an effort to learn more about the client's situation and problems.
12. A properly conducted interview contains three phases: introductory, management, and termination.

REFERENCES

Carkhuff, R. R. & Berenson, B. G. (1977). *Beyond counseling and therapy* (2nd ed.). New York: Holt, Rinehart & Winston.

Collins, M. (1977). *Communication in health care.* St. Louis: C. V. Mosby.

Cormier, L. S., Cormier, W. N., & Weisser, R. J. (1984). *Interviewing and helping skills for health professionals.* Monterey, CA: Wadsworth Health Sciences Division.

Duldt, B. W., Giffin, K., & Patton, B. R. (1984). *Interpersonal communication in nursing.* Philadelphia: Davis.

Elder, J. (1978). *Transactional analysis in health care.* Menlo Park, NJ: Addison-Wesley.

Froelick, R. E., Bishop, F. M., & Dworkin, S. F. (1976). *Communication in the dental office.* St. Louis: C. V. Mosby.

Gorden, R. L. (1980). *Interviewing: Strategy, techniques, and tactics.* Homewood, IL: Dorsey.

Hillman, R. S., Goodell, B. W., Grundy, S. M., McArthur, J. R., & Moller, J. H. (1981). *Clinical skills: Interviewing, history taking and physical diagnosis.* New York: McGraw-Hill.

Murray, R., & Zentner, J. (1979). *Nursing concepts for health promotion.* Englewood Cliffs, NJ: Prentice-Hall.

Rogers, C. R. (1951). *Client-centered therapy.* Boston: Houghton Mifflin.

Sundeen, S. J., Stuart, G. W., Rankin, E. D., & Cohen, S. A. (1985). *Nurse-client interaction—Implicating the nursing process.* St. Louis: C. V. Mosby.

What is it to be wise?
'Tis but to know how little can be known;
To see all other's faults, and feel our own.

Alexander Pope, Essay on Man

9

Learning

Upon completion of this reading and suggested exercises, the student will be able to:
1. Discuss the professional helper's role as a teacher.
2. Define learning.
3. Compare and contrast behavioral and Gestalt field theories of learning.
4. Discuss differences in learning styles.
5. Describe the principles of learning that are fundamental for optimal learning.
6. List and explain the four steps of the teaching process.

All professional helpers have a teaching component inherent in their roles. Although they may not be teachers as such, they are helpers in the learning process. Through their efforts, others are able to learn new knowledge, concepts, attitudes, and behaviors. Like teachers, helpers ask others who have a learning need to take a risk—to trust them. As in any helping relationship, time must be spent proving that trust is warranted. All the principles of helping and communication must be actively utilized so that the learning process can be a pleasant and satisfying one.

THE PROFESSIONAL HELPER AS TEACHER

When does the professional helper teach? You might say that the helper is always engaged in some form of teaching. Much of the teaching is spontaneous, meeting the needs of the client as they arise. Think for a moment about the last time you had blood drawn. The technician probably explained what would happen and why. The technician was able to answer your questions concerning the amount of blood taken and the need for pressure at the site. This kind of teaching is informal and spontaneous, without much time for thought and preplanning. Professional helpers are constantly alert to such opportunities for teaching.

Sometimes helpers find that clients need more formalized teaching. These needs are met by purposely designing a specific class or assignment that will address the needs of the client.

Most of the interactions helpers have with clients involve spontaneous rather than formalized instruction. The teaching that is done is usually outside the classroom and on a one-to-one or small-group basis. Teaching is a very important part of the helper's role, since it is usually the catalyst that is responsible for the client's change in behavior. As this is an extremely critical portion of the helper's role, the helper must be cognizant of learning theories, learning styles, and the learner as a person as well as of various teaching and methodological techniques.

Teaching has frequently been likened to guidance (or counseling), although some authors feel they are definitely different. As professional helpers, we use components of both processes to enhance our client's adaptation. Marriner (1979) differentiates counseling and teaching. She describes the latter method as necessary when a client lacks information and self-direction. The former method becomes more useful as the client becomes more knowledgeable and self-directive. Redman (1976) describes the differences as being mode-oriented. She states, "Guidance, counseling, and support focus on development of attitudes and feelings, whereas the most traditional focus of teaching has been intellectual growth, and training has been thought of as concerned with psychomotor growth" (p. 10). Regardless of one's categorizations and definitions, the professional helper uses all of these components in promoting high-level wellness in the client.

This quest for learning is to some degree a natural one. Studies in human behavior, particularly literature describing the growth and development of people, reinforce this belief. Krause (1970) has described seven categories of the social environment common to all individuals in a way that is particularly pertinent to us as we consider the concepts of teaching and learning. Of these seven categories, three are related to activities in the teaching-learning process. They are as listed:

1. Self-disclosing, in which an individual can appropriately reveal attitudes, opinions, and beliefs to one or more people;

2. Sponsored teaching, which refers to behavior in a social setting, such as a school, in which one person works in ways designed to change or improve the behavior of another;

3. Cooperating or joint working, a social behavior that involves movement toward a mutually recognized goal with some promise of compensation.

These three activities are extremely important to helpers as they begin to devise care plans for their clients. Recall that an atmosphere conducive to trust and disclosure is a basic element of any helping relationship. Similarly, once a learning need is established, cooperation between the helper and the client is necessary if they expect to work together toward a mutual goal.

WHO IS AN EFFECTIVE TEACHER?

What are the qualities and roles of an effective teacher? Some say the effective teacher determines what the learner needs to know and provides the learner with the necessary tools to accomplish this task. Others disagree; they say the teacher guides and directs the learner and it is the learner's responsibility to determine learning needs. The ultimate goal of the professional helper is to have the client decide independently upon learning needs and act accordingly. However, most of us realize that during stressful situations this may often be an unrealistic task. The client needs guidance and direction. This does not negate, however, the fact that learners as well as helpers must be accountable for learning activities. The helper is never solely responsible for making the learner learn! People learn when they are ready—not before.

As with any helper in a relationship, a teacher must be positive and realistic. Self-esteem, self-awareness, and self-understanding are important qualities that all teachers should possess. Recognition and acceptance of one's own strengths and weaknesses are vital. The helper should enjoy teaching and be able to convey that with enthusiasm to the learner. Most importantly, the helper needs to develop a teaching style that is comfortable as well as effective.

The effective teacher should be accepting, supportive, and nonjudgmental toward the learner. As time and positive experiences produce trust in the learner toward the teacher, a friendly environment conducive to learning will emerge. The teacher should be consistent with approach and expectations, but maintain enough flexibility to be able to adapt to the needs and learning styles of clients. This is especially true if children are involved. It is critical, therefore, that the helper be aware of individual and group similarities and differences as relationships develop. Ideally, an effective teacher will be able to so motivate the learner that he or she will not only want to learn, but will develop and maintain an intrinsic desire to learn throughout life. Remotivating someone to want to learn, once initial desire is lost, can be very difficult. Above all, the teacher should show positive regard for those being helped and remember that they are individuals striving for independence. This task is easier if one enjoys the role of helping, understands the clients, and remembers one's own "first experiences." One of the greatest creators of empathy is remembering your own first attempts at learning—your first swimming lessons, first birth or death, hospitalization, first day at school. As a perceptive and stimulating person used to say to her students as they developed into helpers, practice "thereness." When you are with clients, be totally with them. Give them your undivided, individual attention for what time you have, however short.

It is most important for an effective teacher to know the subject matter thoroughly and be able to organize it in a way that is logical and understandable to a learner. Clients should be taught sound problem-solving methods. The differences in meaning that words and experiences have for individuals must be recognized. To be meaningful, new information must relate to something the learner has already grasped or mastered. Certainly it is unrealistic to expect someone to be able to divide numbers if he or she does not yet fully understand multiplication. In order to make learning situations most meaningful, a teacher must start where the learner is by assessing his or her capabilities, limitations, motivation, and styles of learning. Frequent evaluation and open communication will help a teacher to know the learner and his or her progress or lack of progress more accurately. An effective teacher is one who can support and praise students' efforts and work cooperatively with them toward their learning goals. Openness toward others' ideas and creativity in approach and methodology are dual components in successful teaching. Flexibility in manner of presentation is extremely important in meeting a learner's needs. One must view the learning process as a natural one with ups and downs, like all human growth experiences. It needs to be fostered as such, never manipulated. One must recognize that learning needs generally arise from the learner's environment. It is vital that the learner begin to determine what he or she needs to know. A stimulating and creative teacher should be able to encourage the learner to move toward the ultimate goal of independence.

It is important for you, as a beginning professional, to recognize your potential as a teacher. As you capitalize on your abilities and develop teaching strategies, pay particular attention to improving your weak areas so as to enhance your effectiveness. Equally as important is knowing who the learner is and what he or she brings to the situation. What is learning, and how does it affect a person?

LEARNING—WHAT IS IT?

Learning is a process that profoundly influences our lives. Without learning, our ability to grow, to change, and to adapt to the environment would be lost (Fig. 9–1). Simply defined, learning is the "acquisition of information that

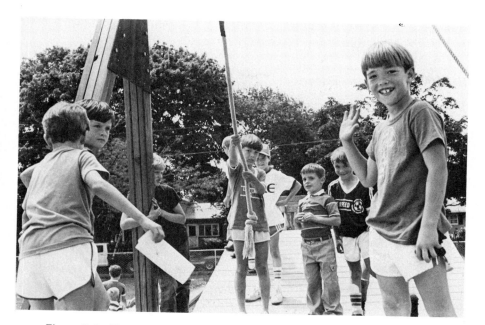

Figure 9-1. Play is a child's work. Done in a nonthreatening environment, it facilitates learning. *(Photo credit to Carolyn Hames.)*

causes a change in behavior" (Rambo, 1984, p. 65). Sometimes the behavior change is obvious—remember the first time you were able to ride a bicycle without training wheels! At other times, however, the behavior change is less obvious—think for a moment of how your attitudes toward your brothers and sisters have changed since you have reached adulthood. In a broad sense, learning means doing or feeling something that you were not capable of previously.

Learning is, then, a change in behavior, attitudes, insights and/or perceptions (Bigge, 1976). Since it is very difficult to measure accurately how much knowledge a person has actually gained, educators often define learning as an observable or nonobservable change in a person's behavior, feeling, or knowledge due to direct or indirect motivation in an active process. To those of us involved in helping professions, learning is a way of enhancing one's level of adaptation to the environment.

THEORIES OF LEARNING

Let us consider the question of how one learns. Although much has been written about theories of learning, it is difficult—in fact, impossible—to simplify and categorize these theories in a way that will meet the approval of all educators and psychologists. At best, we can say that most of the major theories seem to be classifiable into two broad categories: (1) behavioristic, stimulus-response conditioning theories,* and (2) cognitive Gestalt field theories.†

Stimulus-Response Theories

Proponents of stimulus-response theories describe learning as a change in behavior. This theory is commonly associated with Pavlov and his classical conditioning of dogs. Dogs that normally salivated at the presence of meat were taught to associate meat with the tone of a tuning fork. Pavlov discovered that, when he removed the meat, the dogs would continue to associate the tone with eating and salivate when they heard it without the meat being present. His research pioneered work on operant conditioning, in which stimuli either in the form of reinforcement or rewards are given to the learner when something has been satisfactorily learned. The behaviorists have found that behavior changes when the person is "stimulated" in such a way that a certain "response" occurs.

Conditioning can be an effective method of encouraging the learner to behave in an appropriate manner. Teachers often use this approach in an effort to encourage desirable behavior. Think, for example, of the preschool teacher who rings a bell to get the students' attention. Students soon learn that they are to sit quietly when the bell rings.

Sometimes conditioning is used to discourage people from repeating undesirable behavior. Parents often use discipline as a method of conditioning behavior.

> Consider the case of John, a sixth grader. His parents have "grounded" him for 1 month because of his failing grades. If his grades improve, his parents will remove the restrictions. This negative reinforcer (grounding) is introduced to discourage John from failing or, in a more positive sense, to encourage John to bring up his grades.

Stimulus-response theories may at first seem to be a helper's dream. It is relatively easy to learn how to use and to schedule reinforcement. However, as experienced helpers will tell you, sometimes these approaches are not as effective as first hoped. "Reinforcement theory looks upon the learner as a detached intellect" (Tanner & Tanner, 1980, p. 417). By its very nature, stimulus-response learning is mechanical. Students may, in fact, change behavior, but this change may only be short-lived. The weakness in these theories is that they do not encompass the needs of the whole person. Helpers

---

*Including the work of Edward L. Thorndike, John B. Watson, B. F. Skinner, K. W. Spence, O. H. Mowrer, J. M. Stephens, I. Pavlov, and Guthrie Hall.
†Originated in Germany in the early 20th century with Max Wertheimer (1880–1943), Wolfgang Köhler (1887–1967), Kurt Koffka (1886–1941), and Kurt Lewin (1890–1947). Others included are R. Barker, A. W. Coombs, and H. F. Wright.

agree that there are times when this approach is useful, especially as clients learn how to focus on a problem and to solve it. Consider the following example:

> Andrew is an active, playful 5-year-old who is often too busy to do simple tasks such as hanging up his coat after school. His mother decides that Andrew is old enough to hang up his coat and works on a system with Andrew to help him to remember his coat. If Andrew hangs his coat up for 5 days, he is given a special reward, i.e., allowed an extra half hour of television. If Andrew does not hang up his coat on any given day, he is not allowed to watch any television on that day.

Andrew quickly learns that he will be rewarded for hanging up his coat. His mother is pleased with his behavior change and feels that, for this problem, the reinforcement approach was most appropriate.

Stimulus-response theories, however, are not appropriate for all learning situations. These theories seem focused on the behavior of the learner, rather than on the learner as a person. Ultimately, this narrow focus deemphasizes the role of the learner, making it difficult for the learner to develop insight into his or her behavior and to grow and change (Bevis, 1982).

Cognitive-Field Theories

Gestalt or cognitive-field theories emphasize a different approach. The word "field" derives from the belief that teachers work with students who are uniquely interacting with their environment. It is the teacher's desire to help a student reorganize his or her perceptions and understandings of things, ideas, and situations. This is done by exposing him or her to new concepts and experiences and then helping the student relate these to his or her present "field." Consider the same example of 5-year-old Andrew:

> Andrew's mother decides that he is old enough to be able to understand the importance of neatness and hanging up his coat. Together they discuss each other's perceptions of the importance of hanging up your coat. Andrew's mother tries to help him by likening her points of emphasis to feelings to which he can relate.

Gestalt-field theorists emphasize processes and affective goals. "Indeed, the key difference between Gestalt and reinforcement theories is that purposes and motivations are viewed as important to learning by Gestalt theorists" (Tanner & Tanner, 1980, p. 417).

John Dewey (1938) advocated learning by doing. Dewey's belief was that the student must become intimately familiar with the environment, and in doing so learning will take place. Familiarity with the environment and knowing what is expected are definite advantages. The clients not only feel good about what they have learned; they feel an inner sense of competence that affects their whole being.

The Gestalt-field theorists assume a humanistic approach to learning. They emphasize that "motivation for growth toward becoming self-actualized is inherent" (King & Gerwig, 1981, p. 6). They believe that people responsibly evaluate their own behavior and make improvement as deemed necessary. They do not believe that learning occurs by stimuli from the external environment, as the behaviorists do.

> Consider Ed Hughs, a 70-year-old retired businessman. Ed has always wanted to learn to paint. He decided that he now has the time and enrolls in art classes. He is not pleased with his first few paintings, but he keeps reading and listening to his teacher. He notices that, with time and practice, his art work is beginning to look better. He feels a certain satisfaction and pride in his work as he brings it in for his teacher to critique.

As you can see from this last example, Ed Hughs' feeling of accomplishment and self-worth are as important as his actual ability to paint. His development as a person and his ability to self-actualize are of critical importance to his learning.

Remember the history teacher who gave you your choice of final exam questions? You were told to choose three out of five questions and to write your own question if you did not like the teacher's. Once you began the assignment, you realized that it was not as easy as it first seemed, but you were really learning a lot about history. You liked being allowed some flexibility—to determine that content which you would like to study further.

It is probably rare to find a learner—or teacher—who is pure in his or her approach or needs. Most of us, in fact, are eclectic. We may tend to learn better with one approach or another, but most likely we learn by a blending of the two. In teaching, it is the basic style of learning that is most important after all. If the learner's style can be identified, and the teacher can respond with a similar style of teaching, the chances of successful learning are greatly improved.

LEARNING STYLES

Each of you has a slightly different approach to learning—as will each of your clients (Fig. 9–2). "The individual student brings with him distinctive resources for transforming what he studies into knowledge with personal meaning" (Ericksen, 1974, p. 2). It is most beneficial for a teacher to gain some understanding of these resources in order to present new information in a way that will be most helpful for the student.

> The personality characteristics which distinguish one student or group of students from another are often called student learning styles. . . . Such characteristics include a variety of attitudes and values students have about learning, how they like to think, and how they want information presented. (Fuhrmann & Graska, 1983, p. 102)

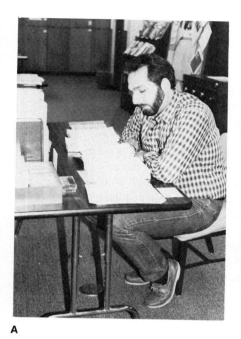 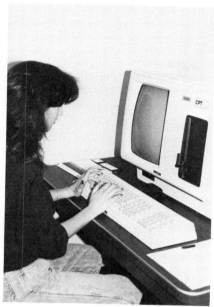

A   B

Figure 9-2. A. Reading continues to serve all of us as a valuable way to learn. **B.** Computer technology is challenging our learning potential. *(Photo credits to Peggy Haggerty.)*

Cognitive aspects of learning styles include such areas as how people solve problems. Styles indicate how people learn and how they process information (Messick, 1976). Some clients find it easier to use inductive approaches, that is, to learn the various parts and ultimately put them together as a whole. Other clients find it more useful to use deductive methods, that is, to study the whole first before examining the various parts that make up that whole.

Witkin (1976) identified two distinctive types of cognitive styles: field-dependent and field-independent styles. It is believed that people develop preferences for one of these approaches. Field-independent individuals rely on organization and structure for learning. These people learn by using an inductive approach: they analyze individual parts and ultimately put all the parts together. Consider the secretary of the student council. This person is responsible for seeing that the meeting minutes are accurate and that each correspondence from the organization is clearly written and distributed to the appropriate people. Field-dependent people have difficulty learning in parts and thus favor deductive methods, that is, studying the whole first before examining the components that make up that whole. This gives them an overall picture to demonstrate how the parts intermesh. Consider the president of the same student organization. This person is responsible for overseeing the entire student council. Although the president may not necessarily understand how the tasks of each group are accomplished, he or she should have a good idea of what the purpose of the student council is and how the council, as an entire group, will affect the student body.

Most people probably use a combination of styles. Learning styles include biophysical and psychosocial as well as cognitive aspects (Keefe, 1979). Some people learn by visual cues; they see a picture or a diagram and can recall the facts. Others learn by listening; they hear certain facts and are able to assimilate these into their knowledge base. Others learn by reading. Most people learn by using a combination of senses.

Psychosocial aspects are, also, important and often unique to each individual. Some of you prefer to "cram" before an exam, while others of you pace your study time. Students who wait until the last minute to study often state that they do better under stress.

How one processes information is only part of one's learning style. Recall that it also includes attitudes and values pertaining to learning. For those who have had positive and successful past experiences with learning, learning may be viewed as challenging and enjoyable. For a client who has not been as fortunate, learning a new skill or behavior may be burdensome or threatening.

It behooves the professional helper to know as much as possible about the client. How does the client feel about learning something from you? Has the client come to this physical therapy session willingly and enthusiastically, feeling that something will be gained, or is the client simply listening to what you have to say because this is part of the hospital discharge plan? Would the client prefer to have you demonstrate crutch walking while he or she listens and watches? Or would the client learn best by viewing an 8-minute video on crutch walking and trying to perform this activity with you as a facilitator? Should you emphasize the individual steps of crutch walking first or start with a broader explanation of what must be learned?

Clearly, the helper as teacher has many things to consider. As you might expect, the helper, too, has a style preference and may find it easier to teach someone who shares that style. Professional helpers, however, must expand their capabilities and methodologies in order to be effective with a variety of clients.

You must remember that clients who have health problems often have difficulty engaging in learning activities. Relying on previous learning styles is not always possible for them, because illness sometimes interferes with the ability to pay attention. Even the most intelligent and well-educated clients will ask for directions to be repeated and for simple explanations.

LEARNING PRINCIPLES

In all learning situations, there are some basic principles that need to be considered. They are as follows:

Readiness

One of the most important facets of learning is readiness. This means that the person is ripe for learning, that the biophysical, psychosocial, and cognitive self are adequately prepared for the learning process. In other words, the person must be physically mature and intact enough to be able to learn a particular skill or concept. Also, the learner must be psychosocially and cognitively mature enough to relate perceptions, experiences, and knowledge and use them to compose new behaviors and ideas. Thus, the growth and developmental functioning of a learner is a critical factor to consider when assessing learning potential.

Physically, the body systems must have the constitutional capacity to function within the limits that will be needed for the desired learning. Most important, of course, is the brain and nervous system, the body's center for learning and organization. Without its crucial biochemical and physical changes, learning is impossible. When psychomotor skills are to be developed, the muscular system must be intact and responsive. Without the use of sight, visual relationships are not possible. Not only must systems be intact; they must be appropriately developed.

The normal 8-month-old, for example, cannot be expected to learn to walk because the child's muscular-skeletal system is not strong enough to support and balance his or her body weight in an upright position. A 6-year-old boy may have the physical ability to hold a pencil in order to learn to write, but if he has never been given the opportunity to develop this fine motor skill, he cannot be expected to write.

Physical readiness is a particular important consideration for health professionals who, by nature of their profession, work most commonly with patients who are motivated to learn because of an actual or potential health problem. Consider a patient who is 2 days postsurgery and has a large abdominal incision.

Because Mrs. Tucker is suffering from stomach problems, she is motivated to learn new health behaviors that will free her from complications. She is ready to learn and, even though she is uncomfortable, she cooperates with the nurse's instructions. It is up to the teacher, in this case the nurse, to determine this readiness and to plan accordingly.

The helper assessing physical readiness must have a keen understanding of human growth and development. Perhaps infant and childhood abilities are the most complex to learn because of rapid maturation during this time. The skilled, experienced helper has at his or her command an accurate knowledge base regarding the physical abilities and inabilities of clients. Certainly, there can be nothing more frustrating than wanting and trying to learn something that is physically impossible for you to do successfully!

Psychosocial readiness is a second consideration. The psychosocial mode involves such things as attitude, feeling, and emotion. Clearly, a person can be physically and cognitively able to learn, but if the concept or behavior is "out of touch" with the person's present way of believing or living, it is of little or no use and, therefore, the person is not ready to learn it. For example:

Karen is a senior in psychology. This is her last semester, and she is trying to write her term paper. Although she has been to the library several times to research her topics, she seems unable to accomplish anything. She is engaged to be married 2 weeks after graduation and is very busy planning a wedding for about 200 guests.

Although Karen has the ability, physically and cognitively, to do her term papers, she is unable to concentrate on her schoolwork because of her preoccupation with her wedding plans. Another example might be an elementary school teacher who, in order to promote classroom harmony, may try very hard to instill a sense of respect for property and privacy in the children she teaches. But a child who has grown up and presently lives in an environment where these values have no meaning is not psychosocially ready to learn them. It is important to realize that this does not necessarily mean the child will not learn these values—only that it will be more difficult to do so because of the negative readiness factor caused by the influence of the subculture.

It is helpful for professionals to have a basic awareness of the motivational tendencies for people from the cultures and subcultures with whom they work. If helpers are alert to the dangers of stereotyping, they can effectively utilize this knowledge as baseline data to be verified or rejected during assessment of the individual's psychosocial readiness. For example, a dietician working with a family from a low socioeconomic group needs to be cognizant of the human tendency to provide for the present before considering the future. In teaching this family about utilization of the four basic food groups, the dietician may need to remain present-oriented rather than include discussion of freezing foods for future consumption.

In addition to having a basic knowledge of group behavior, it is beneficial to know the primary psychological tasks of varying ages. Just as physical abilities must be individually assessed, so must psychosocial characteristics. Erik Erikson (1963), a psychologist, has proposed eight ages of man according to psychological development and maturity. He describes a major developmental task for each of the eight ages, from infancy through senescence. It is Erikson's belief that during each stage a significant amount of energy is expended in working toward resolution of a primary problem. Though this problem may not be resolved totally, it predominates in this stage only and sets the foundation for work in the next stage. If it has not been resolved, subsequent development will be more difficult and time will be "taken away" from the next problem so that work on its resolution can continue. Table 9-1 briefly presents Erikson's theory of psychosocial development. Note that the corresponding ages are not to be considered absolute, but rather as approximations based upon normal maturation.

Lastly, cognitive readiness must be evaluated. This refers to the individual's intellectual, perceptual, language, and creative abilities based on heredity, maturation, and experience.

Billy is a precocious 3½-year-old. He is able to repeat the alphabet forward and backward, print all his letters, and dial the telephone. He has excellent recall of stories and events. Although technically he is not old enough to enter kindergarten, he is ready cognitively.

One of the most widely utilized of the theories of cognitive development was introduced by Jean Piaget, a Swiss psychologist. He proposed that as each person develops cognitively, he or she becomes more intellectually sophisticated and mature. He represents this as a complex progression through four stages of thought, presented in simple form in Table 9–2. Although Piaget correlates specific ages with the stages of cognitive development, the ages he identifies are not as important as the order of the stages.

Motivation

We have seen that a crucial consideration in learning potential is readiness. We have also referred to motivation. Certainly, readiness and motivation may be considered early partners in the process of learning. "Motivation hinges usually on how the learner perceives the value, the meaningfulness, or the instruction for him" (Megenity & Megenity, 1982, p. 170). Motivation is simply the impetus to act and may be either intrinsic or extrinsic.

Intrinsic motivation refers to that internal drive to act in response to a need. It is self-initiated for the purpose of increasing one's adaptation to the environment. "Learning is most effective when an individual is ready to learn, that is, when he feels a need to know something" (Redman, 1976, p. 49). Remember how excited you were about learning to drive a car and how important driver's education classes were?

Extrinsic motivation, considered less desirable, is externally initiated. It occurs when someone else decides you must learn something. Learning that occurs as a result of extrinsic motivation generally takes more effort, concentration, and time. It is classically represented by the familiar classroom scene when the teacher says, "Now, take out your geography books. We are going to learn about Hawaii for your test in 2 weeks." How well we remember the hours spent reading that section of the textbook in which we had no internal interest. Our minds seemed to be always wandering! Thus, learning is most meaningful and most lasting when it is actively sought by and has relevance for the learner (Brunner, 1973; Rogers, 1969). Frequently, extra time spent by the helper developing or stimulating an intrinsic motivation within the learner is time well spent. In traditional teaching settings, we generally begin with extrinsic motivation and hope that it will change to intrinsic as we stimulate the learner to want to learn.

TABLE 9-1. ERIKSON'S THEORY OF PSYCHOSOCIAL DEVELOPMENT

	Trust vs. Mistrust	Autonomy vs. Shame-doubt	Initiative vs. Guilt	Industry vs. Inferiority
8 **Maturity**				
7 **Adulthood**				
6 **Young** **Adulthood** **(18–35)**				
5 **Adolescence** **(13–17)**				
4 **School Age** **(6–12)**				Curiosity, imagination, reasoning skills develop. If successful, growth. If not, failure.
3 **Preschooler** **(4–5)**			Mobility, control, exploration, creativity. Success breeds initiative, failure guilt.	
2 **Toddler** **(1–3)**		Begins to develop self-control. If assertion ac-cepted—au-tonomy. If not, shame, doubt result.		
1 **Infancy** **(0–1)**	Basic needs met —instill trust and hope for future.			

TABLE 9-1. *(cont.)*

Indentity vs. Role Confusion	Intimacy vs. Isolation	Generativity vs. Stagnation	Ego Integrity vs. Despair
			Feel either accomplishment, meaning, satisfaction or dread dying, feel regret, despair.
		Efforts directed towards family, work. If successful, satisfaction. It not, stagnation.	
	Establish basic identity, pursue goals, share self. If unable to find self—isolation results.		
Question identity. Peer group provides security. Experiment with new roles and behaviors.			

TABLE 9-2. JEAN PIAGET'S THEORY OF COGNITIVE DEVELOPMENT

Stage 1 0-2 years old Sensory–motor	Utilizes elementary behaviors to explore his environment. Learns that objectives exist when out of sight (object permanence). In doing so gains a rudimentary concept of space, dimension, quality, and time. Thinking is bound by sensory and motor experiences with beginning imagery and memory. Goal-directed activity with limited alternatives for means of accomplishment emerges. Can assimilate and accommodate.
Stage 2 2-7 years old Preoperational thought	Continues to use language, play, and memory of the past in learning. Begins to repeat relationships between two things, but does not really understand this relationship. Is not able to use the concept of reversibility (that things can change or undergo transition yet remain intact). Uses prelogical thinking as he believes all things center around himself and, therefore, what he experiences and knows, all people should know.
Stage 3 7-11 years old Concrete operations	Can now handle increasingly complex thought problems without having had an actual experience to relate to. Referred to as stage of concrete operations and reasoning. Uses logic and inductive reasoning. Can classify objects by more than one characteristic. Understands conservation concept that things remain the same even if their shape and arrangement are changed. Basically deals with present.
Stage 4 12-15 years old Formal operations	Able to think formally. Can use hypothetical, deductive reasoning about abstract, complex things. Can think internally about situations, propose and test hypotheses, and develop creative ideas. Able to deal with philosophical issues.

(From Piaget, J. (1952). Judgement and reasoning in the child. New York: Humanistic Press.)

Much of our learning, however, is derived from our desire to survive, to be healthy and happy, and to be successful. Much of what we learn and use daily is a direct consequence of intrinsic motivation. In reality, most learning results from a combination of intrinsic and extrinsic motivation (Fig. 9–3). Consider the following example:

Ron has always loved the water and boating. Although he does not know how to sail, he decides to buy a sailboat and learn. His intrinsic desire affords him the impetus to begin to learn to sail independently. He does this by reading books and talking to and watching others. Eventually, however, he recognizes—after a few trial-and-error days at sea—that he has bought a boat too large for him to sail alone. So he goes to the local sailing association to rent a smaller one and discovers that it is their policy not to rent boats to inexperienced sailors. He is required to enroll in a 3-week course of instruction and practice. Thus, his motivation to sail is both intrinsic and extrinsic, and eventually he will be skilled enough to sail his own new boat singlehandedly.

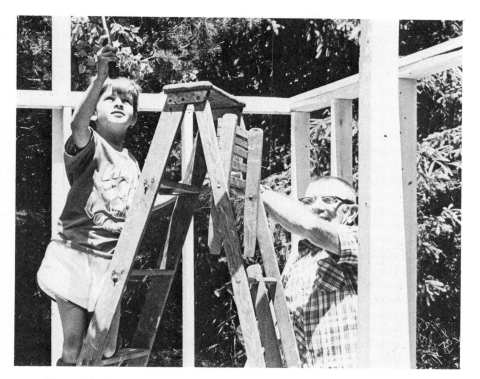

Figure 9-3. The desire to learn is a potent stimulus to human behavior. *(Photo credit to Carolyn Hames.)*

The importance of motivation cannot be overemphasized. In health-related disciplines, helpers may be surprised to learn that formal education often has little to do with success in learning health-related behaviors. Clients who are interested in feeling better are usually motivated to learn as much as possible.

Meaningful Information

In addition to readiness and motivation, a person needs to find meaning and to understand that which he or she is learning. The information should relate to what the learner already knows and proceed from the familiar to the new information, or the unfamiliar (Rambo, 1984, p. 70). How angry we would get as children when our parents made us do something simply because "I said so!" Usually, when they took the time to explain to and reason with us, we performed more willingly, or at least more pleasantly. As Stephens (1965) so aptly states:

If the material is sufficiently meaningful, there may be no forgetting what-ever. As important governing principles, like the old ideas of the conserva-tion of energy, may so help us organize the rest of our ideas that it stays with us for life. Content that is not so brilliantly structured, but which still has much meaning, will be remembered in proportion to its meaning. Non-sense material is headed for extinction before the last syllable is uttered. (p. 210)

If what is learned is truly important to the learner, it will have a lasting impression, as this next example clearly illustrates:

Dan Hunt is a 64-year-old successful businessman who loves to garden as a hob-by. In the late spring, he begins to get the ground ready and plant his seeds. While doing so, he fondly recalls his sixth-grade teacher and the plot of land for which he, as a student, was responsible. How he enjoyed that year! Thus, it was in the sixth grade that Dan first learned how to garden, and at age 64, gardening is one of his greatest pleasures.

A learner needs to understand not only what and why, but how, some-thing will be accomplished. It is not sufficient for a track coach, for example, to prepare young Olympic athletes for competition by only teaching them how to do the pole vault. They also need to be aware of what the record height is so that they will know how they fare in their progress. Similarly, a person who is being advised to lose weight because of high blood pressure needs to know how much weight to lose and needs to have some idea of what would be the ideal weight.

Active Involvement

If learning is to be meaningful and successful, the learner must become ac-tively involved in the learning process. The learner must be free to ask ques-tions, explore new areas, and perform activities. Think about learning the game of baseball. There are many questions a novice player might ask, e.g., "What's the difference between a foul ball and a strike?" or "what happens when you make a double play?" For the athlete, however, truly learning the game means playing the game as well as asking the questions. People must actively engage in the learning process—we do not learn through osmosis. Sometimes this ac-tive engagement is purely mental activity, like studying for a chemistry exam, and sometimes it is physical as well as mental activity, like learning how to drive a car.

Repetition

Repetition is repeating or practicing that which is to be learned. "Studies have demonstrated that 2 to 3 exposures to an idea are necessary before the material will seem familiar or be retained by the learner" (Narrow, 1979, p. 174). Helpers are sometimes hesitant to repeat themselves because they are afraid that they will bore clients. In most instances, however, clients need repetition, as they often do not hear what is being said the first time. Note the following example:

> Gail Janis is using a ski lift for the first time. She listens intently to the directions being given but realizes as she is halfway up the mountain that she is not quite sure how to get off the lift. Luckily, her partner on the lift is experienced, and he explains once again exactly what Gail must do to get off the lift.

Chances are that Gail will need to repeat this skill several times before she masters it. "It is perhaps best to think of repetition . . . merely as a practical procedure ('practice') which may be necessary in order to make sure that other conditions for learning are present" (Gagné & Briggs, 1979, p. 7). A word of caution should be mentioned: Researchers have found that in some situations repetition does not strengthen learning (Ausubel, Novak, & Hanesian, 1978; Gagné, 1977). For example, once a child has mastered tying shoelaces, continuing to practice serves no useful purpose.

Overlearning, or spending additional time on learning behaviors or ideas after they have been mastered, is thought to increase retention, especially when intrinsic motivation is lacking (Figure 9-4). You can probably recall many personal experiences when, while attempting something new, like a tennis stroke, you have said to yourself, "I think I'd better try it just one more time to be sure." Or have you ever studied for a big exam and found yourself going over and over the same page of lecture notes, "just to be sure" you know it? This long-term repetition has little value in learning beyond that of habit fixation (Bevis, 1982). To be of most value, there should be feedback so the learner will recognize mistakes and be able to correct them. Thus, a tennis teacher needs to intervene to tell you how to improve each stroke, or a classmate studying with you needs to change the questions and listen to your answers—to help you improve the review of your notes.

Pacing

"Pacing refers to the structuring of a learning situation by the teacher so that the learner can proceed at his own pace or speed" (Narrow, 1979, p. 176). Pacing is introducing the material at a speed that enables the learner to grasp that which is being taught. This also might be a time when the helper thinks about the style of the learner and whether the inductive or deductive method might be appropriate.

Appropriate pacing of material allows the new information time to "sink in." Assimilation is possible as the learner is able to find the meaning of the new knowledge in relation to what is already known. This enhances true learning, reflection, and insight.

Another consideration is massed versus distributive practice. This refers to the duration of time spent practicing or doing a new behavior or skill. It is generally believed that practice that is spaced over time or distributed is

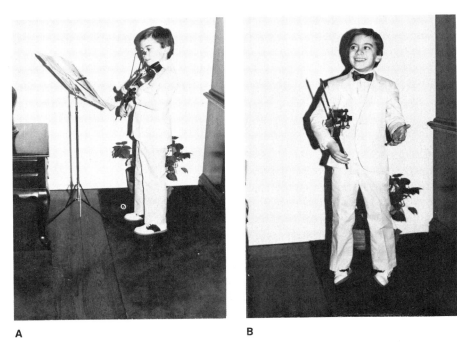

A   B

Figure 9-4. Practice gives one a sense of accomplishment. *(Photo credits to Peggy Haggerty.)*

more productive because it allows time for the learner to reflect on the activity and to rest and rejuvenate energy. Massed practice, on the contrary, encourages boredom, fatigue, and repetition for its own sake.

How frustrating it is to spend a long time desperately trying to learn a skill, only to walk away for a while and then return and do it perfectly! Or remember the last time you had to write a paper or study for an exam. You probably have experienced that feeling of total saturation and loss of concentration and objectivity which follows after hours spent on a single task—not to mention physical discomfort from sitting too long! It is at times like this that most of us find a temporary change of activity and environment beneficial.

Supportive Learning

Once the learner understands what is to be accomplished, the teacher's role changes. It is important that the learner be provided appropriate opportunities to learn. Remember, learning involves risks of success or failure, approval or disapproval, health or illness, and the learner is more apt to take a risk if the teacher provides a secure environment. The learner needs to be able to try new ideas, practice skills, and make mistakes. More importantly, the learner needs to feel a bond of trust with the teacher—needs to feel that the teacher truly wants to help.

Need for Success and Evaluation.   Finally, a learner needs to experience success and to participate in the evaluation of learning. How discouraging it is to try very hard to accomplish something and then fail. Just having someone near to point out the positiveness of your efforts is helpful! The child who is continually told how worthless and slow he or she is may soon lose the desire to try and, worse yet, begin to believe what is said! In helping relationships it is extremely important to provide frequent positive reinforcement so clients know they are learning or appropriately progressing. This might be in the form of a simple pat on the back or a comment, "Gee, you're doing great!" Remember how proud you were when your elementary school teacher put a gold star on your papers, or when your mom hung up on the refrigerator your "masterpiece" of a bird flying over the house—and it did not even look like a bird? Positive reinforcement motivates one to continue to try, to reach, to learn. Concurrent with learning should be constructive evaluation. Because learning involves habit formation, it is far better to stop inappropriate or wrong behavior before it becomes habitual. In the long run the learner will benefit the most by frequent evaluations and honest, open discussions of errors.

Constructive criticism can be very difficult to give and receive if it is not done thoughtfully and tactfully. It is helpful to remember its purpose—to help someone improve that which he or she values and has invested time and effort into creating and doing. It should be done in a supportive, nonthreatening way so as to be received with minimal emotionalism and defensiveness and with maximum objectivity.

In summary, methodologies and strategies of teaching are important but are of little value if the helper does not have a clear understanding of the many facets of learning. Professional helpers devote a great deal of time to teaching and, therefore, need a broad base of understanding.

THE TEACHING PROCESS—FACILITATION OF LEARNING

As facilitators of learning, how do we teach? Regardless of whether teaching is done spontaneously or with advanced notice, it deserves careful consideration and critical thinking. The process of teaching is not unlike the process of systematic problem solving. Teaching, like most things that are logical and comprehensive, has basic steps, or at least a sequential order of occurrences. Although various authors refer to these by different names and terminologies and describe them according to varying theoretical orientations, they are all basically alike in their stripped-down version. For ease in discussion, let's simply call these assessing, designing, interacting, and evaluating.

Assessing	+	Designing	+	Interaction	+	Evaluating	=	Facilitation
Teacher		Environment		Democratic		Feelings		of learning
Learner		Objectives		Flexible		Process		
Situation		and		Meaningful		Learning		
		content				attainment		
		Approach						

Assessing

Once a need for teaching has been initially recognized, three components must be assessed—the teacher, the learner, and the situation. The people involved must recognize and accept their own needs, capabilities, limitations, and potentials. It is frequently helpful to do this via informal discussion, since it will promote acquaintanceship and trust formation. The learner has an opportunity to verbalize those things he or she feels most strongly about and is in most need of learning. The teacher can express his or her degree of comfort and ability to meet identified needs of the learner. Together they can agree—at least tentatively—on the scope of the situation so that both have a mutually shared idea of what needs to be accomplished.

Many college professors do this during the first day of class, when time is spent making introductions and talking about what will be accomplished during the semester. Although teachers differ in style and degree of depth, many welcome students' comments, suggestions, and ideas in this initial meeting. Some professors rely more on verbal exchange, while others use handouts of course information and student questionnaires. In a college classroom situation, some initial assessment has occurred long before the teacher and students meet. It can be expected that the professor has a given amount of expertise, capability, and potential by virtue of his or her faculty status. The students have all met minimal requirements upon admission to the university. By enrolling in a particular course, they have publicly demonstrated a need for particular learning, although they may be extrinsically motivated!

> Mrs. Ellis is a 60-year-old patient suffering from high blood pressure and fluid retention. She is on medication to help alleviate both of these problems, but Sally (her doctor's office nurse) knows that medication alone will not eliminate the problem. Sally spends some time talking with Mrs. Ellis about her health and determines that she is receptive to learning more about ways to increase her adaptation. Sally determines that Mrs. Ellis has a fair degree of knowledge already. They agree that some reinforcement and new information from Sally will enhance Mrs. Ellis's adaptation. They plan to meet the next afternoon.

Designing

This begins as a refinement of the initial assessment and may, in fact, occur so directly that it appears to be simultaneous. For many teachers, it is the most time- and energy-consuming step of the whole teaching process. This is where those initial ideas and assessments are molded and organized. Purposes are clarified, and measurable learning objectives (both intermediate and ultimate) are established. These define behaviors or accomplishments that should be present if learning has occurred.

Content to be taught is prepared, and creative methodologies selected. These may be in the form of small group discussions, lecture, demonstration, or audiovisual presentations. Learners may be engaged in physical activity, as in a laboratory setting, or they may be asked simply to listen or observe. Whatever method is chosen, the environment must be conducive to the development of intrinsic motivation and the process of learning. Specifics like ventilation, furniture arrangement, lighting, and sound are carefully considered to provide the best physical setting.

In college classrooms, most of this is done long before the start of each semester. Last-minute changes, deletions, and additions may be made after the professor and students begin to work together. This degree of flexibility varies with situations and teachers. Certainly, there should be enough room for give-and-take so that rigidity does not interfere with learning.

Sally and Mrs. Ellis both have done some anticipatory thinking before their meeting. They both create in their mind some ideas of what will be accomplished. Specifically, Sally reviews what she knows about high blood pressure and fluid retention. She decides to meet with Mrs. Ellis in a small conference room that is equipped with comfortable furniture and a variety of audiovisual supplies. She plans to talk with Mrs. Ellis about her general response to anxiety and stress and her diet. When Mrs. Ellis arrives, Sally shares her plans. Through discussion, they agree that Mrs. Ellis is a calm, easygoing person who does not seem to have a stress-related health problem. In talking about her diet, however, Sally discovers that it is very high in sodium. Together they determine that Mrs. Ellis needs to follow a salt-restricted diet. They establish some simple objectives. Given a gram scale and new information, Mrs. Ellis will (1) identify foods high in sodium, (2) limit her sodium intake to 1 gram/day, and (3) weigh herself daily and report any gain over 6.6 kilograms to the nurse.

Interacting

Although there usually has been some personal interaction by this time, *interacting* refers to the exchange that occurs when content is presented to the learner. For learning to be most successful, content must be organized and presented in such a way that the learner can relate to it. It must be meaningful and understandable to the learner. Guiding learning in a democratic atmosphere with questioning and discussion rather than strict telling will enhance the quality of interaction. So will supportive, nurturing behaviors that encourage creativity and independence. Intermediate objectives should be continually evaluated and redefined as necessary. Demands for independent problem solving should be minimized until the student has grasped the essential material. Feedback should be critically constructive and consistent. In all situations, the basic principles conducive to developing and maintaining helping relationships should be employed.

Compare your own past experiences in education. Think about a particular professor whom you liked and respected and in whose class you felt you did well and learned effectively. Why? What was the interaction like? How did it differ from another you can recall when learning did not occur? As you strive to become an effective helping teacher, begin to develop and incorporate some of the qualities displayed by those you find most helpful.

> Mrs. Ellis and Sally begin to implement their design. Sally has Mrs. Ellis write a nutritional history of all the things she has had to eat and drink in the last 48 hours. With the aid of a filmstrip on low-sodium diets, Mrs. Ellis is able to determine the amount of salt she consumes in her present diet and review the foods and fluids high in sodium content. Together, they plan several menus favorable to Mrs. Ellis's taste that are within the allotted sodium restriction. Mrs. Ellis is weighed, and her blood pressure is taken for baseline data. Encouraged, Mrs. Ellis agrees to see Sally the following week and bring a weekly nutritional history with her at that time.

Evaluating

This final step involves several components. Since the goal of any learning situation is to increase one's capabilities toward adaptation, we certainly need to evaluate the learning attained. This is based on previously established learning objectives. But perhaps equally as important is the process and tone of the interaction. How did things go? What were the participants' reactions and attitudes? What about the smoothness of the process? It is most helpful if these are evaluated as the relationship is occurring, so that the need for change can be recognized and dealt with early. Evaluation of the process should be as objective as possible, with subjectivity retained for evaluation of feelings. If intermediate and ultimate objectives have been comprehensive and well constructed, they can be invaluable during evaluation. In the end, we should have a realistic picture of what went well and what did not go as well in the teaching-learning process and interaction.

As a college student, you will probably be involved in evaluations, both verbal and written, at the end of courses. Occasionally, there is sharing at midpoints in the semester. This is usually of learning attained (in the forms of quizzes and exams!) rather than of the process and feelings. Ideally, evaluation should be of all three components in an ongoing manner.

> When we finally see Mrs. Ellis and Sally, they are evaluating the progress of the previous week. Mrs. Ellis has restricted her sodium intake but can still identify areas for continued improvement. She has weighed herself daily. They agree for her to keep a nutritional history for one more week and meet with Sally at least one more time before she becomes more independent.

CONCLUSION

Thus, we have seen that teaching is an intricate part of helping. The teaching-learning period is a time and opportunity for clients to change, to grow, and to become independent. While it demands responsibility and accountability from the teacher, it survives solely on the readiness, desirability, and efforts of the learner. As Kahlil Gibran so appropriately states in *The Prophet* (1965): "He [the teacher] does not bid you enter the house of his wisdom, but rather leads you to the threshold of your own mind. For the vision of one man lends not its wings to another man" (p. 56).

IMPORTANT REMINDERS

1. Learning is a process that helps us to grow, change, and adapt to our environment.
2. Stimulus-response learning theories are useful when helping clients to change behavior.
3. Gestalt or cognitive-field theories emphasize the learning process and affective goals. These theories stress that feelings of accomplishment and self-worth are an important part of the learning process.
4. Helpers must be cognizant of various learning styles and present new information in a manner that is congruent with the client's learning style.
5. Readiness, motivation, meaningful information, active involvement, repetition, pacing, supportive learning, and success are learning principles that each helper needs to remember when engaging in a learning situation with clients.

REFERENCES

Ausubel, D. P., Novak, J. D., & Hanesian, H. (1978). *Educational psychology: A cognitive view* (2nd ed.) New York: Holt, Rinehart & Winston.

Bevis, E. O. (1982). *Curriculum building in nursing* (3rd ed.). St. Louis: C. V. Mosby.

Bigge, M. L. (1976). *Learning theories for teachers.* New York: Harper & Row.

Brunner, J. S. (1973). *The relevance of education.* New York: Norton.

Dewey, J. (1938). *Experience and education.* New York: Macmillan.

Eriksen, S. C. (1974). *Motivation for learning: A guide for the teacher of the young adult.* Ann Arbor: University of Michigan Press.

Erikson, E. H. (1963). *Childhood and society* (2nd ed.). New York: Norton.

Fruhrmann, B. S., & Grasha, A. F. (1983). *A practical handbook for college teachers.* Boston: Little, Brown.

Gagné, R. M. (1977). *The conditions of learning* (3rd ed.). New York: Holt, Rinehart & Winston.

Gagné, R. M., & Briggs, L. J. (1979). *Principles of instructional design.* New York: Holt, Rinehart & Winston.

Gibran, K. (1965). *The prophet.* New York: Knopf.

Keefe, J. W. (1979) Learning style: An overview. In *Student learning styles. Diagnosing and prescribing programs.* National Association of Secondary School Principals.

King, V. C., & Gerwig, N. A. (1981). *Humanizing nursing education—a confluent approach through group process.* Wakefield: Nursing Resources.

Krause, M. S. (1970). Use of social situations for research purposes. *American Psychologist, 25,* 753–8.

Marriner, A. (1979). *The nursing process—a scientific approach to nursing care.* St. Louis: C. V. Mosby.

Megenity, J. S., & Megenity, J. (1982). *Patient teaching: Theories, techniques and strategies.* Bowie, MD: Robert J. Brady.

Messick, S., et. al. (1976). *Individuality in learning.* San Francisco: Jossey-Bass.

Narrow, B. W. (1979). *Patient teaching in nursing practice—a patient and family centered approach.* New York: Wiley.

Piaget, J. (1952). *Judgement and reasoning in the child.* New York: Humanistic Press.

Rambo, B. J. (1984). *Adaptation nursing assessment & intervention.* Philadelphia: Saunders.

Redman, B. K. (1976). *The process of patient teaching in nursing* (3rd ed.). St. Louis: C. V. Mosby.

Rogers C. (1969). *Freedom to learn.* Columbus, OH: Merrill.

Stephens, J. M. (1965). *The psychology of classroom learning.* New York: Holt, Rinehart & Winston.

Tanner, D., & Tanner, L. N. (1980). *Curriculum development* (2nd ed.). New York: Macmillan.

Witkin, H. A. (1976). Cognitive style in academic performance and in teacher-student relations. In S. Messick et al. (Eds.), *Individuals in learning.* San Francisco: Jossey-Bass.

Men see little, presume a great deal, and so jump to conclusions.
John Locke

10

Problem Management

Upon completion of the following reading and suggested exercises, the student will be able to:
1. Define the basic needs of the person according to Maslow.
2. Define actual and anticipated problems and explain their relationship to need satisfaction.
3. Discuss factors that influence one's perception of needs and problems.
4. Name and describe five different ways of handling problem solving.
5. Analyze a personal problem, using the scientific method of problem solving.
6. Identify skills and behaviors of the helper that facilitate problem solving with a client.
7. Discuss the implications of solving problems by the use of research.
8. Identify the purposes of research.
9. Discuss the qualities necessary in the helper that foster research.
10. Define the phases of assessment, planning, implementation, and evaluation, and relate this problem-solving process to the profession he or she plans to enter.
11. Write objectives and interventions, using behavioral terminology.

As students of a helping profession you are in the process of learning to work with people more effectively. Although the people with whom you work may differ greatly in age, education, degree of health, and independence, all of them have in common their humanness and their need for help. For a variety of reasons they are faced with problems that they cannot independently resolve. As a helper it is your responsibility to assist these clients to increase their adaptation and to solve problems independently.

Since all problems (whether overt or covert) ultimately stem from unsatisfied needs, the professional helper must have a thorough understanding of people. Problem solving as presented here is an organized process based on satisfaction of human needs. Only when a need cannot be or is not being met does a problem exist.

BASIC NEEDS OF MAN

Generally, needs are defined as those physiological or psychological requirements that are essential for survival. One of the people who has contributed significantly to our general understanding of the theory of basic needs is Abraham Maslow (1954). He viewed man as a universal, holistic being. In his book, *Motivation and Personality*, he describes all people as different but with basic universal needs. He identifies five basic categories of need as follows:

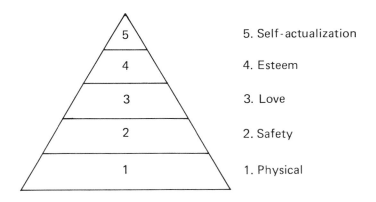

5. Self-actualization

4. Esteem

3. Love

2. Safety

1. Physical

In the first category Maslow describes the primary needs of all people for physical requirements of living: food, water, rest, oxygen, and sexual fulfillment. Because these are generally necessary for survival, they are the base for all others and normally dominate in priority.

Secondary to the physical requirements are safety needs. These include reasonable freedom from threat, orderliness, predictability, rituals, rules, and laws. They provide a degree of structure and stability to the external environment so that one is more likely to successfully adapt to it. Love needs include a sense of belonging. Unlike sexual drive, love is an inner feeling of affection, of caring for and being cared about.

Beyond love is self-esteem—the "free to be you and me" syndrome. Feeling good about one's self and one's role increases self confidence, and in turn, respect for others.

Last is the need for self-actualization or self-fulfillment. It is perhaps the most frequently unfulfilled need of them all. It is a feeling of having accomplished all that one is capable and desirous of doing.

Maslow did not intend for these needs to be rigidly pursued, one category after another. Rather, like human development, there is a general order of progression that allows for partial fulfillment of several categories at a time.

BARRIERS TO NEED FULFILLMENT

There may be times in a person's life when pursuit of higher-level needs is not realistic because more primary needs are unmet. For example, it is unlikely that a prison inmate would have much opportunity to be rehabilitated or prepared for successful, productive community living if only physical and safety needs are being met. The inmate cannot be expected to "go straight" and have positive feelings about him- or herself if others have not allowed opportunities for the inmate to at least partially meet love and self-esteem needs.

Illness also can pose a barrier to need fulfillment. Perhaps one of the most difficult things for health-care professionals to do is to try to help patients feel a sense of pride and accomplishment when they are physically ill. Fulfillment of physical and safety needs can demand a great deal of time and energy expenditure. This is particularly true when the physical limitation is permanent, chronic, or seemingly endless in the patient's perception. When you are ill, it can be very depressing and self-defeating to try so hard to accomplish the things you are used to accomplishing with ease when you are well. Similarly, it can be very difficult to adapt to life when you have, for instance, lost a leg or had a colostomy. Health care workers, therefore, need to help patients simultaneously fulfill needs at varying levels.

PERCEPTION OF PROBLEMS

This raises an important issue, which is that problems are a matter of perception (Fig. 10–1). Frequently what seems to be a problem to one person is not perceived that way at all by another. Certainly you can recall a time when a friend perceived a situation as catastrophic and you felt it was of minor significance! Similarly, perceptions change within a person at different times and in different situations. Remember the last time you were getting ready for a big date, only to discover a large red blemish right in the middle of your cheek? A somewhat devastating occurrence to an adolescent, who tried every

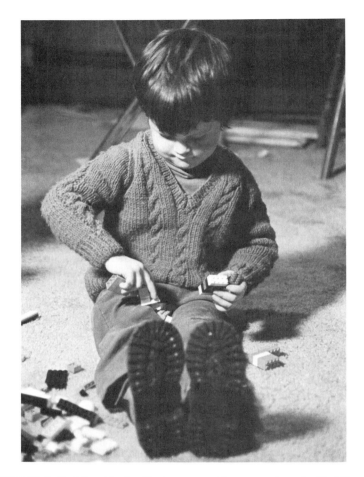

Figure 10-1. Building blocks, like human problems, are viewed with different perceptions and rarely have only one solution. *(Photo credit to Steve DeRosa.)*

cover-up technique imaginable to diminish the problem! Yet as this same person earlier in the morning stood with a younger brother in the kitchen making chocolate chip cookies, it was totally insignificant! It is not uncommon for the magnitude of problems to change in different situations. Similarly, time can seemingly diminish or increase the magnitude of problems. A good night's sleep—while not a professional helping technique—can be very refreshing to one's perception of the situation.

It is critical that helping professionals convey a feeling of respect for their client's perception of a problem. Many of the nontherapeutic things we do and say to clients stem from a lack of empathy and respect for the client's viewpoint. It is expected that, as helpers, we are able to assess the situation more objectively since we are outside of it. Therefore, one of our primary goals is to help a person more clearly and rationally examine the situation. Frequently, with understanding and a feeling of support from the helper, the client feels less threatened and more capable of thinking about constructive alternatives in problem solving.

NARROWING THE PROBLEM

Another factor that is beneficial to a client's problem-solving ability is to limit the complexity of the situation. Unfortunately, clients are often confronted with several problems simultaneously, thus increasing the complexity of the entire process of problem solving. This can be overwhelming and lead to difficulty in focusing on a specific part of the problem situation. The client may not even know where to begin to solve the problem. When this happens, it is helpful for the helper and client to identify each component of the problem separately and to list these singular problems in order of priority. These can further be distinguished as actual and anticipated problems.

Generally, actual problems are those that are current and in most immediate need of solution. Anticipated problems are those that do not yet exist or are temporarily being handled, but the potential for their needing solution in the future is expected.

There are some specific factors that should be considered when determining which problems are in most immediate need of solution:

1. Which problems are most threatening to physical and mental functioning? Certainly those that are life-threatening need to be handled first.
2. What is the client's perception of the actual and anticipated problems?
3. What is the helper's perception of the actual and anticipated problems?
4. What is the available time frame within which solutions can be achieved? In some situations, the quality of the problem solving is directly related to the time available to spend on it.

PROBLEM-SOLVING METHODS

Once needs and problems are determined, how are they solved? Probably each of us uses a number of different ways to handle our everyday problems. Francis (1967) has described five methods of problem solving:

1. *Unlearned, inherent problem solving*—determined largely by biological endowment, not by thought; approaches problem in fixed, blind ways; exemplified in the animal kingdom.
2. *Trial-and-error problem solving*—occurs with no forethought or perception of relationships, but simply by means of chance and process of elimination.

3. *Insight problem solving*—solution occurs originally by trial and error, but during or after the situation one has a limited ability to see the relationship and thus the reasons for solution; may be repeated again if same exact situation presents itself.
4. *Vicarious problem solving*—uses imagination to visualize the situation and predict consequences based upon assumptions. The chance of error in the actual situation is decreased if assumptions have been correct. This method of problem solving necessitates an ability to use language and conceptualize ideas.
5. *Scientific-method problem solving*—characteristic of Western civilization's orderliness, efficiency, and refinement; uses logical thinking, going from the parts to the whole with six steps: (1) defining the problem, (2) collecting data, (3) formulating an hypothesis, (4) evaluating the hypothesis, (5) testing the hypothesis, and (6) forming conclusions.

Modification of the Scientific Method

It is imperative that helping professionals use a sound theory base and a systematic approach to problem management. Thus, the scientific method is frequently used as a foundation for effective problem solving. It helps to organize facts, ideas, and judgment. Since this particular method was developed for use in the pure sciences, a modified form is needed for application to the human sciences. The following is a systematic approach to problem management in a helping relationship:

1. Recognize and define problem.
2. Gather and assess information.
3. Develop alternative actions and probable outcomes.
4. Select specific actions and plan implementation.
5. Implement action.
6. Evaluate action and outcome.

Analyze a simple everyday task—dressing yourself—in terms of this problem-management model. First, you must begin with a need. Since it is cool, fall weather and you have been invited to go horseback riding in the morning, you decide to plan what you will wear. You have a physical need for warmth and a safety need to protect your legs from chafing. When you look in your closet, you find only skirts and wool dress slacks. At this point you recognize a barrier to fulfilling your need. The problem is that you do not have anything in your closet that is appropriate to wear horseback riding tomorrow morning. In order to help you decide what to wear, you call your friend Sue, who tells you she is wearing her riding pants and that you will probably grab a quick lunch at a local hamburger stand. You again look through your closet. The laundry bag reveals two pairs of dirty blue jeans. You realize that you are presently wearing a pair of heavy beige corduroy pants. It is Thursday, and you remember that the stores are open late. You also realize that your friend Janice is next door and she wears the same size pants as you do. Having gathered this information, you begin to formulate some ideas:

Action	Probable Outcome
1. You could go to the store and buy something.	You would diminish your already limited financial resources. You might not find something appropriate that fits. A trip downtown would take time you had planned to use studying.
2. You could wear the same pants you presently have on, since they are fairly clean and are of heavy material.	You would not look as clean and fresh as you like to. You could stain the legs of your beige pants by rubbing against the horse.
3. You could wear something in your closet.	You might ruin a pair of wool slacks by going horseback riding in them. Your legs would be directly against the horse if you wore a skirt.
4. You could borrow a pair of heavy, dark-colored slacks from Janice.	You would feel obligated to lend something to Janice if you borrowed from her. Her slacks might not fit as well and as comfortably as you like. You would feel badly if anything happened to her slacks while you had them.
5. You could wash your dirty clothes at the laundromat.	A trip to the laundromat would take time you have planned to use studying. You would be wasting money because your laundry bag only has four dirty articles of clothing in it.
6. You could wash one pair of dirty blue jeans by hand in the sink.	There is a possibility they might not air-dry by morning.

Once you have thought of all your alternatives, you select what seems to be the most reasonable solution. You decide to forego the studying tonight and take a trip to the laundromat to wash your blue jeans. You will simply switch what you had planned for tomorrow night's activity (writing a letter home) with studying because it is easier to write in a noisy laundromat than it is to concentrate on studying. You decide that the amount of money you waste on a wash load is worth the physical comfort and the good feeling you will have about your appearance tomorrow. You prepare to implement your decision by readying your laundry, money, soap powder, stationery, car keys, and coat. You tell your roommate where you are going and drive to the laundromat. On your way home you realize that it is earlier than you had thought it was and that you finished the whole letter. The next day as you wait for Sue to pick you up, you have an inner feeling of looking good and knowing that you are dressed appropriately and are going to enjoy the day.

Remember that in the beginning of this discussion it was indicated that this represented management of a simple everyday problem. How complex it appears! And daily this is done scores of times!

EFFECTIVE PROBLEM MANAGEMENT

In thinking about problem solving it is important to keep in mind that it is a dynamic process allowing—and in fact encouraging—flexibility. It systematically lends direction but does not dictate it. At any point it is possible to reverse direction and return to a former step.

Effective problem management is a learned process that has the capability of improving with experience, growth, and development. While at first it may seem slow and laborious, speed and efficiency are usually gained. Parts or individual components of the process soon become whole. In time, the process becomes second nature and we do it "without thinking." As professional helpers, responsible and accountable to a person who may be temporarily dependent and is counting on our skill and assistance, we cannot let this happen. It is imperative that we approach each client and situation with an open mind and our undivided attention, lest we gloss over the process and, in doing so, shortchange the client. Experience and expertise will, however, enable professionals to move through the problem-management process with more finesse and speed. Those of you new to the helping role will probably find it necessary at this point to examine the process and consider each component separately and at length.

A key to effective problem solving lies in the first step. Too frequently we rush over this and think we know what the problem is, only to determine later that we were working in the wrong direction. It is wise to keep the assumed definition of the problem flexible while gathering and assessing data so that it can be validated or changed as needed. For optimal effectiveness it is absolutely necessary to have an accurate problem statement before alternative actions are designed.

Accurately defining the problem statement can be confusing when a situation presents itself with multiple problems superimposed upon one another. When this happens it is necessary, as previously discussed, to sort problems out from one another. Professionals can usually help clients do this because they are less emotionally involved in the situation and, generally, have a more objective perspective. Similarly, problem management can be frustrating when there appear to be countless possible solutions. As a professional helper, you may find times when your client can only deal with one or two immediate problems or solutions, but you can do some anticipatory handling of others. This can save a great deal of time, which is a valuable asset, especially during crisis situations. With experience, professional helpers gain skill and expertise in handling increasingly complex problem situations. It is wise for the beginning helper to avoid working with clients who have an accumulation of complex problems. Ethically, each professional helper must consider, with each prospective client, if the assumed responsibility is more than can be effectively handled.

RESEARCH IN THE HELPING PROFESSIONS

Your ability to solve problems is crucial to the growth of your profession and, more importantly, to the care of your clients. Helpers are continually asked to solve problems, and it is an expectation that research—a scientific approach to problem solving—will be used. Most of you probably have the idea that research is only for the scientists—not for the people, such as nurses, pharmacists, teachers, etc., who have direct contact with clients needing professional services.

As you become a more experienced helper, you will learn that no one has a better appreciation, feel for, and understanding of the client than those helpers who work in practice settings. These are the professionals who best know common needs and problems. Certainly, the scientists can be of assistance, but the most important person in identifying researchable questions involving client needs is you—the professional helper!

At this point in your career, most of you are anxious to help people by actual "hands-on" experience. You want to see, to talk, to teach, to help, and to minister to clients. You want to get to know the client's environment and to feel comfortable in that setting. Successful researchers know the client thoroughly. You are encouraged to get a lot of experience in helping before you become a researcher. You might even decide that research is not one of your interests—which is fine. Not all helpers have to be researchers. However, all helpers have to have an understanding of the research process and to keep abreast of research findings in their field as well as related fields. Remember, research is the scientific approach to solving problems. It is proof to the world that rational solutions work.

What Is Research?

Most of you are already familiar with research and how the findings can be used. Television, newspapers, and even advertisements routinely bombard us with research findings. How have most of you learned about the importance of fluoride in toothpaste? Or low cholesterol in the diet? Or not smoking to avoid lung disease? Meteorologists use research findings to study and report weather findings. Psychologists use research findings to learn about such diverse issues as birth order and psychosomatic illness. Homemakers use research findings when they cook. Have any of you ever tried altering a recipe by changing the liquid, type of shortening, or baking powder? It may turn out fine—but if it does, it is by chance. We are given certain guidelines to follow because researchers have learned through systematic investigation that recipes are better when specified amounts of ingredients are added.

Research, then, "is a scientific process of inquiry and/or experimentation that involves purposeful, systematic and rigorous collection of data" (Dempsey & Dempsey, 1981, p. 4). Once the data have been collected, they are analyzed, and interpretations are made. These findings either expand our existing knowledge of the topic or represent new knowledge areas. Research is the discovery of something new. It is an orderly attempt to find answers to problems.

The term *research* is often used incorrectly. As students you talk about doing research for a paper. In actuality, you are doing a literature review and writing a term paper. This is very different from doing a research project. In the former case you are merely communicating knowledge that already exists—your intention is not to find a new answer or solution to a problem (Dempsey & Dempsey, 1981).

Purpose of Research

Seaman and Verhonick (1982) state that "the purpose of research is to observe in order to know; to know in order to predict; to predict in order to control; to control in order to practice and prescribe in a professional manner" (p. 5). Simply stated, the purposes of research are to describe, to predict, to control, and to prescribe.

Observation.   Those helpers who are doing research to learn more about a situation are involved in descriptive and/or exploratory studies. These studies are based on the helper's or the researcher's ability to observe the environment. Note the following example:

> The highway department has been assigned the task of resurfacing three major roads. The decision of which three roads to pave comes after several months of observing major traffic patterns. The city planner has reported to the town council that 90 percent of the traffic travels on these three roads and that the roads are in need of repair. These roads lead to the freeway; thus, the planner feels that they will continue to be used.

It was this researcher's responsibility to describe the traffic patterns, conditions of roads, and potential continued usage. Without this kind of study, less appropriate roads might be chosen for repair. Thus, accurate objective description was vital in this situation.

Prediction.   Prediction is a second purpose of research. Your predictions suggest that certain relationships exist among the factors being studied. In the helping professions most, if not all, of our predictions are associational rather than causal. For example, we cannot determine that the death of a parent *causes* stress in the middle-aged adult. There are too many other factors that influence the adult. But we can determine that the death of a parent is *associated* with stress in the middle-aged adult. Note:

> Mary Snodgrass, aged 45, is a working mother of three teenage daughters. She is an account executive who has been divorced for 10 years. Her mother's recent death means not only the loss of a loved one but the added burden of straightening out the mother's business affairs, selling the family home, and caring for her aging father.

It is difficult to know which of these factors causes Mary's stress and how much each is contributing to her stress. We can determine, however, whether or not the death of a parent is a factor that is associated with stress in this middle-aged adult, Mary Snodgrass.

Information that enables us to predict client problems or behaviors is important because it allows helpers to recognize cues. If we know through research that situation B usually follows situation A, for example, then as helpers we can prepare ourselves and our clients.

Control.   As you begin to know your environment and to predict what will occur, you will be ready to move to a third purpose of research—control. This means that you will be able to exercise some authority over the various factors that influence clients. As a helper in any number of disciplines, you will learn that certain interventions will promote positive responses for the client. Note:

> Arron Jones, a 40-year-old Vietnam War veteran, is seen weekly for physical therapy. Rob Jacques, the therapist, knows that Arron is in a great deal of pain and that exercise enhances that pain. Mr. Jacques decides to try meditation before the treatment to see if pain will be alleviated. In a sense, he is adding a control to the client's environment. Something—in this case, meditation—is being introduced to the client in an attempt to alleviate pain. If Mr. Jacques learns that meditation is successful with Arron, he will prescribe that this be done before all of Arron's treatments.

Prescription.   The fourth purpose of research, prescription, is an outcome of research and is "based on the fact that the goal to be achieved is a desirable one" (Seaman & Verhonick, 1982, p. 6). It also should be understood that Mr. Jacques did not choose meditation out of "thin air." He has done extensive reading and has learned that several researchers have found this technique successful.

This form of research involves experimentation. Mr. Jacques has read several research studies involving the use of pain medication versus the use of meditation in alleviating pain in patients with chronic disabilities. Scientists must prove through research which approaches to care they can prescribe. We can no longer let our intuition rule our practice—as professional helpers, we need to study the appropriateness of our interventions scientifically.

Research Problems

As you learned earlier in this chapter, it is helpful to narrow the focus of a problem before attempting to solve it. Research problems are no different from the problems discussed earlier—they, too, must meet the factors established to determine priority. Defining the research problem is thought to be the most difficult step in research. Learning to narrow the focus of the topic and then to state the problem clearly is an art that sometimes takes a long time to accomplish. The more clearly and accurately the problem is stated, the greater the chance for satisfactory conclusion.

"The development of a research problem is essentially a creative process, dependent upon imagination, insight and ingenuity" (Polit & Hungler, 1983, p. 64). As stated previously, the researcher must be familiar with the topic being studied. The more knowledge the person has, the easier it is to state the problem. As you have probably surmised, there are lots of problems around for helpers to solve. Helpers should be extremely cautious when deciding upon a problem to study, for time and energy can be wasted on problems that truly do not address problematic areas for patients. For example, a study that investigates the use of square versus rounded bed corners could easily be designed. However, the knowledge generated from this study would have little, if any, relevance to a client population.

Hence, the problem must be *significant*—meaning that if it is studied, it will benefit the client or the community, or contribute to theoretical knowledge. The problem needs to be researchable; the factors or variables must be defined clearly and precisely. Furthermore, the researcher has to determine if it is feasible to do the study. Time considerations, subject availability, facilities, money, ethics, and researcher experience are all important factors in determining the feasibility of the study.

Qualities in the Helper That Foster Research

Although scientists, doctorally prepared professionals, and college professors may best understand the technical aspects of research, it is truly the helpers at the "grass-roots" level who generate ideas for research. Those who contribute most successfully to the research endeavors of their professions seem to possess certain qualities. The following qualities have been adapted from Diers' (1979) discussion of the qualities inherent in researchers. They are as follows: inquiry, relatedness, insight, and appreciation.

Inquiry, or curiosity, is almost inherent in novice helpers. You are enthusiastic about learning everything. Many of you will quickly begin to ask why problems happen and will wonder how problems can be solved. Researchers have an insatiable quest for inquiry—they can never know enough.

Relatedness helps the researcher put problems into their proper perspective. By observing repeated incidents over a period of time, the researcher begins to determine which problems are of real significance. "To see a problem as a possible research problem, one must be able to make mental connections between incidents and cases" (Diers, 1979, p. 11). Compare the following examples:

> Erika Jones babysits for two boys, aged 4 and 2, from 3 to 7 P.M. She notes that they both become cranky at about 4:30 P.M. and are difficult to manage until they eat dinner at 5:30 P.M.
>
> Ellen Smith is a teacher who has worked in several nursery schools in different parts of the country. She reports that mothers of 2 to 4-year-olds continually complain that their children are irritable in the late afternoon. This irritability seems to cease after they eat dinner. Many of her teaching colleagues report similar complaints.

Both observations are essentially the same. However, Erika Jones is reporting data on an isolated incident, while Ellen Smith is reporting data on repeated findings over several years. In this example, it would be reasonable to derive a research question from the second example because several mothers throughout the country are reporting similar behaviors in 2 to 4-year-olds.

Insight, or having the inherent ability to analyze a situation critically, is very important. Sometimes when helpers have been working in one place for a long time, they do not see all that is happening. The helper becomes oblivious to subtle changes. A person who is less familiar with the environment can often contribute by sharing initial thoughts about what is happening. Note the following example:

> Mrs. Durrigan, an eighth-grade teacher, is complaining that her social studies students are experiencing the "end-of-the-year slump." She tells Ms. Ellis, the student teacher, that this is a usual occurrence and she just lets students bide their time until the year ends. "Lots of good students lose their grades—they just give up."
>
> Ms. Ellis, however, does not agree with Mrs. Durrigan. She notes that the homework assignments and tests have been much harder during this part of the semester. There seems to be a real push to finish the text. The students appear "stressed" rather than "bored."
>
> She discussed this observation, and Mrs. Durrigan agrees that perhaps she has increased the work load. They both feel this should be investigated further.

Hence, it sometimes takes "a new pair of eyes to see research possibilities" (Diers, 1979, p. 11).

The researcher must always maintain an *appreciation* for those professionals who practice in clinical settings. On the one hand, new people viewing a situation can be very helpful; but, on the other hand, you must always listen to the comments and observations helpers with years of experience make regarding issues in their practice. Experience often brings wisdom to the situation. A seasoned helper may have little, if any, knowledge about techniques of research, but may have developed several innovative ways to help clients. Consider for a moment:

> Sally Hooper has had 15 years of experience as a nutritionist in a large metropolitan community agency. She is orienting Elsie Smyth, a new dietician, to the agency. Sally tells Ms. Smyth that she always considers the client's life-style and economic status before planning the diet. She candidly mentions that medical condition is less important than she was taught in school. "Clients who don't want to follow a diet or who can't pay for foods on the diet do not comply with the dietary regime!"

Sally Hooper has made a very interesting and important observation. She may, in fact, have the key to giving advice to clients. Without realizing it, Sally Hooper has the makings of an excellent research proposal. Researchers must listen to and watch professionals who practice, for the practice setting is the research arena.

It's All in the Question

"The term research means to search again, to take another, more careful look, to find out more" (Selltiz, Wrightsman, & Cook, 1976, p. 4). In taking this new, more careful look, the researcher carefully scrutinizes the situation and asks pertinent questions. These questions are of fundamental importance to all of us, for in the question lies the strength of the proposal.

A researchable question is one that yields hard facts to help solve a problem, produce new research, add to theory, or improve practice (Brink & Wood, 1983). Research questions must be relevant to issues and needs of clients and helpers. The questions need to be stated concisely and clearly. Research questions fall into one of three categories or levels (Brink & Wood, 1983; Diers, 1979). It should be remembered that these levels are merely used to classify types of research. They are not intended to evaluate the quality of research approaches— level 1 is as important as level 3.

"First-level questions are exploratory in nature, examining new areas of insufficient knowledge" (Brink & Wood, 1983, p. 12). Research in the level 1 category is useful because it generates new information and new insights. This approach to research addresses "What is this?" kinds of questions. Such studies are undertaken when the researcher needs to describe a given pheno-menon or situation.

> Consider for a moment the researcher who is interested in nurses' reactions and responses to patients who attempt suicide. The researcher is unable to find any information in the literature regarding nurses' reactions to suicides. Thus, the question, "What happens when nurses interact with suicidal patients?" is asked. The answer to this question will be in descriptive form after careful, in-depth analysis of data collected from interviews with nurses.

Second-level questions focus on the relationships between two or more variables previously described but never studied before (Brink & Wood, 1983, p. 12). These studies address the "What is happening here?" type of questions (Diers, 1979). The researcher is attempting to determine if one factor is related to another factor. There is an attempt to show relationships. Causality, how-ever, is not a goal of this kind of study.

> Consider the following question: What is the relationship between self-concept and success in college? In asking this kind of question, the researcher must find that there is a relationship between students' self-concepts and their academic achievement in college. It may be that those students who feel most positive about themselves make better grades. If so, there may be a relationship.

Third-level questions are useful in predicting that one variable influences the other in a certain way (Brink & Wood, 1983). Questions asked at this level require in-depth knowledge and ask, "Why does this relationship exist?" These types of research questions build upon the findings of either first- or second-level research questions. They also lend themselves to experimental design that can lead the research to the eventual goal of prescription. Note the following example:

> Laurie Jones, a nurse with several years of experience, feels that diabetic patients should be instructed in diabetic foot care before they leave the hospital. Although patients are told about the care, they are not given any formalized instruction. Many of the diabetics return with severe infections in their feet. Laurie designs a research study in which she compares the rate of infection between two groups of diabetic patients—one that has formalized instruction and one that does not. If Laurie learns that the group of patients with instruction has less infection, she can institute a new policy that all diabetics must have special instruction regard-ing foot care in her agency.

Thus, Laurie has demonstrated that one variable influences the other.

Research, then, is one approach to problem solving. It also is used to generate new information and insights, and when used in this way is not a comparison of alternatives, but more of an undifferentiated search within specific problem areas (Fox, 1982). As evident by the past discussion, research is an absolute necessity for growth of the helping disciplines.

NURSING PROCESS—AN EXAMPLE OF PROFESSIONAL PROBLEM SOLVING

There are many other examples of problem solving that assist helpers to organize their thoughts and services clearly. One profession that has made remarkable progress in accomplishing this in recent years is nursing. Through implementation of the nursing process (a practical application of the scientific method), nurses have made great strides in more accurately, effectively, and efficiently defining and resolving patients' health care problems.

Table 10–1 demonstrates the relationship between the modified scientific method of problem solving, the research process as previously described, and the nursing process.

The nursing process is "an orderly, systematic manner of determining the client's problems, making plans to solve them, initiating the plan or assigning others to implement it, and evaluating the extent to which the plan was effective in resolving the problems identified" (Yura & Walsh, 1978, p. 20). Thus the nursing process model involves the phases of assessment, planning, implementation, and evaluation—not unlike the phases of a modified scientific method. Let us consider some special points of interest about each phase. As you read, think about how this process might be applied to other professions.

Assessment

The assessment phase of problem solving is perhaps the most crucial because it involves accumulation of pertinent, accurate data with sufficient scope and depth on which to identify patient needs and determine barriers to need fulfillment. This is done both verbally and nonverbally through observation of the patient's behavior. The nursing history is particularly helpful in that it is an organized series of questions designed to obtain specific information about a patient. Ideally, a nursing history is taken on admission to the hospital or health care facility. If obtained by a skilled professional, the nursing history and interview can help initiate a trusting relationship between the client and the nurse. The nurse gathers necessary data, and the client feels that individuality is respected and that care necessary for the client's well-being will be provided.

The final step of assessment occurs after the data base is accumulated. From the collected data and the nurse's theoretical knowledge, patient needs are established and listed by priority.

Theories such as Maslow's help to determine which of the patient's needs are most important, and therefore must be met first. Remember, whenever

TABLE 10-1. COMPARISONS OF SCIENTIFIC METHOD, RESEARCH PROCESS, AND NURSING PROCESS

Modified Scientific Method	Research Process	Nursing Process
1. Recognize and define problem	1. Define the problem; narrow scope; focus on importance	Meet patient, take patient history; review other data about patient, including medical history and medical diagnosis
2. Gather and assess information	2. Background—study observations and literature	Assess data; review nursing theory and medical information; identify problem areas; establish nursing diagnosis
3. Develop alternative actions and probable outcomes	3. Research design—implement a methodology, a way to study the problem	Develop realistic, measurable patient objectives; consider alternative means to accomplish these objectives
4. Select specific action and plan intervention	4. Study the findings; do they allow you to prescribe certain treatments?	Develop written nursing care plan with specific nursing interventions; communicate via Kardex, patient's chart, and team and/or individual conferences
5. Implement action	5. Evaluate, refine, and continue to question and conduct research	Begin nursing interventions, provide patient care; document in nursing notes; communicate in team and/or individual conferences
6. Evaluate action and outcome		Evaluate and terminate helping relationship (discharge or transfer patient). Return to Step 2 as needed for continuation or modification of action

possible, the patient is expected to engage actively in the problem-solving process by defining needs. Using keen judgment and sensitivity, the nurse then draws conclusions about why the stated needs are not being met. This difference between what should be and what is, combined with a judgment of why, creates a *nursing diagnosis*. Nursing leaders are now in the process of formulating lists of nursing diagnoses and nursing nomenclature. After nursing diagnoses are determined, planning commences.

For example, Tom is being admitted to the hospital because of a bladder infection. The nurse begins to ask some questions and observe his behavior. During the brief interview, Tom makes several negative comments about himself. All of them relate to the fact that he is an amputee and, therefore, less of a person than others. As part of the assessment, the nurse concludes that one of Tom's problems involves his self-image. The nurse states a nursing diagnosis as "Alteration in body image secondary to recent amputation of left leg."

Planning

The planning component involves development of a nursing care plan. For each nursing diagnosis, patient objectives or behavioral outcomes are stated, and alternative approaches are developed and selected. Patient objectives serve as guidelines or directional markers, signifying in specific, realistic, measurable terms behaviors that will be observed in the patient if problems are resolved. They are stated in terms of the results that are intended to be achieved. They are specific and measurable, so that progress can be readily identified and evaluation simplified. An important component of creating realistic objectives is the time factor, as there certainly must be enough time to accomplish that which is desired.

In a profession such as nursing, objectives serve to organize activities and unify the reasons for individual action. When each member of the helping team is aware of the objectives that are being sought, there is more likely to be sharing of ideas regarding approach to nursing care. This reduces the chance that each member in the health team will intervene in an independent manner, thus preventing the outcome of continuity of care.

Writing Behavioral Objectives

There are several guidelines that can be followed in learning to write behavioral objectives. According to Mager (1972), each objective should include the following criteria:

1. A statement of the desirable overt behavior that the patient will demonstrate if the objective is successfully accomplished. This is a single, observable, measurable activity or ability that is the expected outcome or end product of effort. As such, it is a positively worded statement of what will occur rather than a negative statement of what will not occur. It should be stated clearly enough to avoid misinterpretation. This is usually easier to do for physical than for psychosocial behaviors.

2. An indication of the circumstances or conditions under which the behavior is expected to occur. These may name allowable aides or equipment, or specify known restrictions or methods.

3. A specification of the criteria of acceptable performance or success. This is a description or standard by which the patient's performance will be evaluated.

Becknell and Smith (1975) suggest that to these three components be added the subject as a specification of who or what is expected to demonstrate the desired behavior. They furthermore suggest that it is not always necessary to name all four components, specifically the conditions and criteria. Conditions may not be relevant, and criteria may be extraneous or implied in the behavior. In most situations, however, patient objectives will include a statement of the subject, behavior, and criteria.

At this point an analysis of some examples of patient objectives may be helpful. Remember from Chapter 1 that there are three modes or areas in which assessment of clients is done: biophysical, psychosocial, and cognitive. Consider the following examples of patient objectives in each of the modes:

Cognitive Mode.   Within two days, Sally will correctly demonstrate crutch-walking technique using a three-point gait.

- Subject—Sally
- Expected behavior—Will correctly demonstrate crutch-walking techniques
- Conditions—Using a three-point gait
- Criterion—Within two days

Biophysical Mode.   The mucous membrane of the mouth will remain smooth, moist, and intact.

- Subject—Mucous membrane of the mouth
- Expected behavior—Will remain smooth, moist, and intact
- Conditions—None
- Criterion—None

Psychosocial Mode.   Before going to the operating room, Mr. H. will discuss his feelings about surgery with the nurse.

- Subject—Mr. H.
- Expected behavior—Will discuss his feelings about surgery with the nurse
- Conditions—None
- Criterion—Before going to the operating room

Once clearly stated objectives for patient behavior are identified, the final step in the planning phase is to determine ways to accomplish what is desired. At this point, teamwork may be helpful, following the old adage, "Two heads are better than one." Whenever possible, the patient and family should be included when objectives are defined. Alternative approaches should consider the patient's resources and capabilities as well as limitations. Once alternatives are determined, those whose outcomes seem more expedient and probable are selected and communicated to everyone involved. Nurses usually accomplish this verbally via end-of-shift reports and periodic team conferences, and in writing via the nurse's progress notes, a part of the patient's medical record. A shortened, quick, reference form of the most crucial interventions and information is usually written in the nursing Kardex (an index and card-type file of daily nursing care requirements). Teachers usually accomplish this via lesson plans and student conferences. Physical therapists, dental hygienists, pharmacists, and other health care professionals often accomplish this by directly communicating verbally with the client, helping the client to decide which objectives are essential.

In most cases the professional has more expert knowledge than the client about a particular problem, and it is essential that the helper share that knowledge during this phase. For example, the dental hygienist explains to the patient carefully why flossing and massaging gums are crucial to a healthy oral cavity. The professional, however, can only share information and offer assistance to the client. Ideally, the client makes the ultimate decision of whether or not to accept a stated objective.

Writing Interventions

Effective written communication of specific approaches chosen can be very difficult. It is frequently easier to do something yourself rather than explain to others how to do it. Because people on the health care team are frequently of varying educational and developmental abilities, it becomes crucial for nursing orders or interventions to be written in clear, concrete terms that are not likely to be misunderstood or misinterpreted.

Becknell and Smith (1975) have established four components to writing nursing orders that help eliminate the possibility of confusion or error. They are:

1. The *behavior* to be performed by the reader or designated individual. This is written in specific, overt terms whenever possible, avoiding the more vague, covert actions (i.e., talk rather than encourage).
2. The *recipient* of the action. This is usually the patient, but it could be a particular part of the patient, like a left thigh or another family member. This may be implied, and therefore not specifically stated.
3. The *object* describing what is to be given, handled, etc., or how the behavior is to be performed. The object may be unnecessary at times.
4. The *frequency* or specific time at which the overt action is to occur.

Again, some examples related to the previously stated objectives may help to clarify these components.

Cognitive Mode.   Show and explain to Sally three-point gait crutch walking On 3/18.

- Behavior—Show and explain
- Recipient—Sally
- Objective—Three-point gait crutch walking
- Time—On 3/18

Biophysical Mode.   Brush teeth with toothpaste and rinse mouth with clean water after each meal.

- Behavior—Brush and rinse
- Recipient—Teeth and mouth
- Objective—Toothpaste and clean water
- Time—After each meal

Psychosocial Mode.   After completion of preoperative teaching, allow 15 minutes to discuss with Mr. H. how he is feeling.

- Behavior—Discuss
- Recipient—Mr. H.
- Objective—Feelings about surgery
- Time—For 15 minutes after preoperative teaching

Interventions may be multidirectional. Ultimately, they should support higher levels of adaptation. This may be accomplished by adding, removing, modifying, or counteracting stimuli; protecting or removing the individual from the stimulus and its effects; and supplementing, modifying, minimizing, or correcting the effects of adaptive responses that are deficient, excessive, or inappropriate.

Implementation

In the implementation phase, nursing action is initiated. Simultaneously, observation of the results, efficiency, and effectiveness of nursing care are noted. An increasingly important part of this observation and critical thinking is written and verbal documentation. In most clinical situations, progress notes regarding accomplishment of the client's behavioral objectives are written at least every 8 hours. Teachers and counselors often keep anecdotal records that document their clients' progress.

One of the most difficult tasks of writing meaningful progress notes is to write them clearly and concisely, making each word "say something." This is a very difficult task for most beginning professionals, and it takes a great deal of effort to develop such a skill. It is most helpful to remember to *describe* rather than *interpret* the behavior that is observed. In other words, progress notes should be objective and factual rather than subjective and commentary. Words like "good," "fair," and "small" should be avoided, since they have multiple interpretations. In addition to what you see, hear, smell, and feel, you should chart those things that you do for or to the client and the client's responses to such care. Nurses' notes as well as other anecdotal records should be a continual record of the client's care and progress. With the recent increase in the number of malpractice cases filed against nurses and other health care helpers, accurate, comprehensive documentation has become vital. After care has been given and documented, final evaluation occurs.

Evaluation

The evaluation phase is a time for reassessment of the client and progress or lack of progress toward the stated objectives. It is one of the most valuable steps of the process, but unfortunately is too frequently slighted. Rarely do people take the time to consider why successful objectives were, in fact, successful. More frequently they make decisions about modifying actions that are not working well. Ideally, evaluation should produce information about objectives that need to be terminated, continued, and/or modified. Included as final written evaluation are the client's discharge notes and transfer notes. These are summations of the client's status and care, designed to give another health care worker a brief but comprehensive review of the client's experience while being cared for in a health care facility.

Remember that evaluation should be occurring throughout the problem-solving process as well as at the conclusion. This allows for immediate modifications to be made. Evaluation at the conclusion of the problem-solving process should include summarization of what has occurred as well as the results of any previous evaluations.

CONCLUSION

We have seen, by closely examining one helping profession's use of problem-solving techniques, that problem solving is a very highly organized system interdependent upon proper functioning of all its components. Although the nursing care process has been used as an example, much of its operation is directly applicable to other helping professions. In any area where helpers are working with clients who are depending upon them, they have a responsibility to assess, plan, implement, and evaluate astutely. Whether done by teachers or dental hygienists, an accurate data base and theoretical expertise are basic. Creation of clear, realistic objectives that later serve as guides to evaluation of what is accomplished have become necessities for optimal helping. Creativeness and flexibility of approach with prompt, accurate documentation is an asset to professional helpers whose major responsibility is to relate effectively with other human beings.

The process of effective problem management, although seemingly laborious and complex, can be easily learned by beginning helpers. By bringing some organization and logic to a problem situation, frustration and needless energy expenditure can be diminished.

IMPORTANT REMINDERS

1. Professional problem management is an organized, learned process that is implemented as needed to help clients increase their adaptation. It is

based on the six steps of scientific problem solving.

2. Although all people have universal needs, perceptions of these needs differ. To facilitate problem solving, it is imperative that there be agreement on the presence of a need and the definition of the problem.
3. Problem solving is most effective when there is an accurate problem statement, clear behavioral objectives of what is to be accomplished, and flexibility of approach with continual evaluation.
4. Research is a scientific approach to problem solving.
5. The purposes of research are to describe, to predict, to control, and to prescribe.
6. Researchers should possess the following qualities: inquiry, relatedness, insight, and appreciation.
7. In the helping relationship, mutual designing of behavioral objectives and planning for intervention between client and helper will foster trust and efficiency of problem management.
8. Professional problem solving involves the four phases of assessment, planning, implementation, and evaluation.

REFERENCES

Becknell, E., & Smith, D. (1975). *System of nursing practice: A clinical nursing assessment tool.* Philadelphia: Davis.

Brink, P. J., & Wood, M. J. (1983). *Basic steps in planning nursing research, from question to proposal* (2nd ed.). Monterey, CA: Wadsworth Health Sciences Division.

Dempsey, P. A., & Dempsey, A. D. (1981). *The research process in nursing.* New York: Van Nostrand.

Diers, D. (1979). *Research in nursing practice.* Philadelphia: Lippincott.

Fox, D. J. (1982). *Fundamentals of research in nursing* (4th ed.). Norwalk, CT: Appleton-Century-Crofts.

Francis, G. (1967). This thing called problem solving. *Journal of Nursing Education, 6,* 27–29.

Mager, R. (1972). *Preparing instructional objectives.* Palo Alto, CA: Fearon.

Maslow, A. (1954). *Motivation and personality.* New York: Harper & Row.

Polit, D. F., & Hungler, B. P. (1983). *Nursing research principles and methods* (2nd ed.). Philadelphia: Lippincott.

Seaman, C. H., & Verhonick, P. J. (1982). *Research methods for undergraduate students in nursing* (2nd ed.). Norwalk, CT: Appleton-Century-Crofts.

Selltiz, C., Wrightsman, L. S., & Cook, S. W. (1976). *Research methods in social relations* (3rd ed.). New York: Holt, Rinehart & Winston.

Yura, H., & Walsh, M. (1978). *The nursing process: Assessing, planning, implementing, evaluating.* New York: Appleton.

Appendix I

Activities

Playing the games and participating in the activities suggested in this section will enhance the learning of the concepts presented in the text. Note that specific exercises are listed for each chapter, although most can be used for a variety of concepts. We suggest that you familiarize yourself with all of them and make decisions about which ones will best suit your needs. It is certainly not necessary to participate in all the suggested exercises; choose those that appeal to your sense of adventure and/or focus on particular areas that are of importance to you. We encourage you to create your own exercises or adapt these as necessary. Have fun!

Adaptation

1. LETTER AND ASSESSMENT

Read the following letter and follow the directions. An example and explanation of a grid response is in Appendix II, p. 265. *Caution:* Participants should *not* read Appendix II.

January 24, 1986

Dear Student,
    My name is Dayle Joseph, and I am one of your classroom teachers. I

consider myself to be a healthy 35-year-old female. It is, generally, with enthusiasm that I welcome students to a new semester. Unfortunately, I am feeling "out of sorts" today and thought you might be able to help me.

You see, yesterday I left work early to do some shopping. I was using my brand-new car. I was looking forward to today because I thoroughly enjoy meeting new students and I like to teach. My mood was quite cheerful as I entered a little store in Wickford. Ah, Wickford—such a pretty place, especially in the snow!

Well, Wickford's not so great when your car won't start. In fact, it's damn ugly. You see, there are no indoor phones—they are all located on the street. Calling the car repair service was not too bad. I figured the battery needed recharging and I'd be off! Waiting, however, for the repair service to arrive was another story. It was cold—real cold. My hands and feet had that all-too-familiar tingling feeling. I was afraid to wait in the stores, because I might miss the repair truck.

At last he came—the day was saved, or so I thought. The man almost smiled when he told me it was the electrical system, not the battery. He made a wonderful diagnosis—leaving me with a car to be towed.

Back to the phones. My feet were freezing in the snow (why didn't I wear warm boots?). My hands hurt every time I dialed the phones. The phone lines were busy. I ran out of change. I began to feel frustrated and exhausted. Today was supposed to be an early day. I had been in the cold for 3 hours.

My sense of humor was lost. My level of adaptation became dangerously low. All my energy had been taxed. Finally, I arrived home, only to realize that I had left all information for today's lecture in my car!

It would be most helpful if you assessed my situation, identifying stimuli that influenced my behaviors. Also, feel free to talk about actual and potential behaviors that you noted. In doing this, carefully consider the biophysical, psychosocial, and cognitive modes. Maybe this type of grid will help you.

Mode	Stimuli	Response	Behavior

Thanks for your assessment.

Your grateful teacher

2. SELF-APPRECIATION EXERCISE

This exercise was designed by Ronald Adler and Neil Towne. It can be found in *Looking Out/Looking In—Interpersonal Communication*, 3rd ed. (New York: Holt, Rinehart & Winston, 1981, p. 82).

As a means of demonstrating the self-appreciation that can come from recognizing that you are growing, do the following:

1. Form a circle in your group. Your group size may be the class as a whole or several small groups.
2. Each group member in turn should complete the following statement: "I'm a long way from being perfect at ＿＿＿＿＿ , but I'm slowly getting better by ＿＿＿＿＿ ."

Here are some examples:

"I'm a long way from being perfect at <u>my job</u>, but I'm slowly getting better by <u>taking on just one task at a time and persisting until I finish.</u>"

"I'm a long way from being perfect at <u>approaching strangers</u>, but I'm slowly getting better by <u>going to more parties and once in a while actually starting to talk to people I don't know</u>" (Adler & Towne, 1981, p. 82).

Discuss how it feels to talk about your strengths? Your weaknesses? Is it more difficult for you to discuss strengths or weaknesses? Discuss your answers with the group.

Culture

1. HOLIDAYS

The purpose of this exercise is to help you "get in touch" with some of your cultural values. As a group, take a moment to share with one another your family traditions on a holiday such as Thanksgiving, Easter, or Independence Day. Be specific as to who participates, what you do, what you eat, the time devoted to various activities, where you go, and so on.

As you share this information, note the reactions of the group members. Do they respond verbally? What do their facial expressions tell you about their responses? How do you feel about their supportive and their surprised responses?

As others are sharing their traditions, think about your response to them. Are you surprised by their experiences?

Openly discuss as a group your feelings and ideas about what has been shared. What implications does this have for professional helpers?

2. CHOOSE THE IDEAL MATE

This exercise, designed by Hames and Joseph, will help you recognize some of your attitudes and values.

It is the year 2001, and you must give the computer your requests regarding the specifics of the mate that you will eventually choose. The information that is needed includes:

- Weight
- Height
- Skin color
- Hair color
- Eye color
- Ethnic origin
- Personality characteristics
- Religion
- Political affiliation
- Socioeconomic group
- Level of education
- Occupation

Please describe the above statistics as honestly as you can. (Disregard those of your present boyfriend, girlfriend, or spouse.)

Look at your answers. Do they tell you anything about your value system? Did you choose a mate who had religious, political, and ethnic affiliations similar to yours? If so, why? If not, why? Did you feel more strongly about some traits than others? If so, which ones did you definitely want to incorporate into the choice of your future mate? Can you tell why you chose the traits you did?

If you are doing this exercise as a group, share your answers to the questions. Compare your answers with those of others. What does this demonstrate about the values and prejudices that people have?

3. ON THE VARIOUS MEANINGS OF WORDS

The following exercise is a shortened version of the one developed by Stewart L. Tubbs and Sylvia Moss in 1974, published in *Human Communication: An Interpersonal Perspective* (New York: Random House).

Column A lists words commonly used in a particular American subculture. Try your luck at matching the meanings found in Column B with Column A.

Column A   **Column B**

_____   1. Blade   1. The best
_____   2. Busted   2. Good
_____   3. Bread   3. Squeal
_____   4. Boss   4. Look over carefully
_____   5. Cop out   5. Really fine
_____   6. Freeze   6. Be genuine
_____   7. Choice   7. Money
_____   8. Heavy   8. Stop
_____   9. Checkout   9. Knife
_____ 10. Come outa your act   10. Caught by police

Discussion

Note how many of the words have infiltrated American culture. Note that some words have different meanings for different cultural groups. Identify words or expressions that have private meanings in your particular cultural group.

Note: The correct answers are in Appendix II, p. 267.

4. WHEN THE FAMILIAR IS NOT SO FAMILIAR

The following game is adapted from one titled "This Is My Nose," developed by Andrew Fluegelman in *More New Games!* . . . *and Playful Ideas from the New Game Foundation* (Garden City, N.Y.: Doubleday, 1981, p. 27).

Try changing the meanings of words and body parts with a group of unsuspecting people. For example, enter a room, point to your nose, and say, "This is my eye." Note the responses of others. Do they laugh? Do they look at you in disbelief? When they respond, point to your leg and say, "This is my head." What happens? Keep going, identifying familiar body parts with unfamiliar terms.

Discuss how you feel when the group responds to you. Do you feel people are laughing at you, making fun of you, or attempting to understand what you are doing?

5. BAFA BAFA

This is a cross-cultural simulation designed by R. Gary Shirts in 1977. For information concerning this game write to: Similie II, 218 Twelfth Street, P.O. Box 910, Del Mar, California 92014; or Navy Personnel Research and Development Center, c/o Department of the Navy, San Diego, California 92152.

6. NACIREMA CULTURE

The following is a description of Nacirema culture as first described by Horace Miner in "Body Ritual Among the Nacirema" (*American Anthropologist* 1956, 58:3, 503–507). After reading this description, answer the questions at the end and discuss as a group.

> Professor Linton first brought the ritual of the Nacirema to the attention of anthropologists twenty years ago (1936:326), but the culture of this people is still very poorly understood. They are a North American group living in the territory between the Canadian Cree, the Yaqui and Tarahumare of Mexico, and the Carib and Arawak of the Antilles. Little is known of their

origin, although tradition states that they came from the east. According to Nacirema mythology, their nation was originated by a culture hero, Notgnihsaw, who is otherwise known for two great feats of strength—the throwing of a piece of wampum across the river Pa-To-Mac and the chopping down of a cherry tree in which the Spirit of Truth resided.

Nacirema culture is characterized by a highly developed market economy which has evolved in a rich natural habitat. While much of the people's time is devoted to economic pursuits, a large part of the fruits of these labors and a considerable portion of the day are spent in ritual activity. The focus of this activity is the human body, the appearance and health of which loom as a dominant concern in the ethos of the people. While such a concern is certainly not unusual, its ceremonial aspects and associated philosophy are unique.

The fundamental belief underlying the whole system appears to be that the human body is ugly and that its natural tendency is to debility and disease. Incarcerated in such a body, man's only hope is to avert these characteristics through the use of the powerful influences of ritual and ceremony. Every household has one or more shrines devoted to this purpose. The more powerful individuals in the society have several shrines in their houses and, in fact, the opulence of a house is often referred to in terms of the number of such ritual centers it possesses. Most houses are of wattle and daub construction, but the shrine rooms of the more wealthy are walled with stone. Poorer families imitate the rich by applying pottery plaques to their shrine walls.

While each family has at least one such shrine, the rituals associated with it are not family ceremonies but are private and secret. The rites are normally only discussed with children, and then only during the period when they are being initiated into these mysteries. I was able, however, to establish sufficient rapport with the natives to examine these shrines and to have the rituals described to me.

The focal point of the shrine is a box or chest which is built into the wall. In this chest are kept the many charms and magical potions without which no native believes he could live. These preparations are secured from a variety of specialized practitioners. The most powerful of these are the medicine men, whose assistance must be rewarded with substantial gifts. However, the medicine men do not provide the curative potions for their clients, but decide what the ingredients should be and then write them down in an ancient and secret language. This writing is understood only by the medicine men and by the herbalists who, for another gift, provide the required charm.

The charm is not disposed of after it has served its purpose, but is placed in the charm-box of the household shrine. As these magical materials are specific for certain ills, and the real or imagined maladies of the people are many, the charm-box is usually full to overflowing. The magical packets are so numerous that pepole forget what their purposes were and fear to use them again. While the natives are very vague on this point, we can only assume that the idea in retaining all the old magical materials is that their presence in the charm-box, before which the body rituals are conducted, will in some way protect the worshipper.

Beneath the charm-box is a small font. Each day every member of the family, in succession, enters the shrine room, bows his head before the charm-box, mingles different sorts of holy water in the font, and proceeds with a brief rite of ablution. The holy waters are secured from the Water Temple of the community, where the priests conduct elaborate ceremonies to make the liquid ritually pure.

In the hierarchy of magical practitioners, and below the medicine men in prestige, are specialists whose designation is best translated "holy-mouth-men." The Nacirema have an almost pathological horror of and fascination with the mouth, the condition of which is believed to have a supernatural influence on all social relationships. Were it not for the rituals of the mouth, they believe that their teeth would fall out, their gums bleed, their jaws shrink, their friends desert them, and their lovers reject them. They also believe that a strong relationship exists between oral and moral character-istics. For example, there is a ritual ablution of the mouth for children which is supposed to improve their moral fiber.

The daily body ritual performed by everyone includes a mouth-rite. Despite the fact that these people are so punctilious about care of the mouth, this rite involves a practice which strikes the uninitiated stranger as revolting. It was reported to me that the ritual consists of inserting a small bundle of hog hairs into the mouth, along with certain magical powders, and then moving the bundle in a highly formalized series of gestures.

In addition to the private mouth-rite, the people seek out a holy-mouth-man once or twice a year. These practitioners have an impressive set of paraphernalia, consisting of a variety of augers, awls, probes, and prods. The use of these objects in the exorcism of the evils of the mouth involves almost unbelievable ritual torture of the client. The holy-mouth-man opens the client's mouth and, using the above mentioned tools, enlarges any holes which decay may have created in the teeth. Magical materials are put into these holes. If there are no naturally occurring holes in the teeth, large sec-tions of one or more teeth are gouged out so that the supernatural substance can be applied. In the client's view, the purpose of these ministrations is to arrest decay and to draw friends. The extremely sacred and traditional character of the rite is evident in the fact that the natives return to the holy-mouth-men year after year, despite the fact that their teeth continue to decay.

It is to be hoped that, when a thorough study of the Nacirema is made, there will be careful inquiry into the personality structure of these people. One has but to watch the gleam in the eye of a holy-mouth-man, as he jabs an awl into an exposed nerve, to suspect that a certain amount of sadism is involved. If this can be established, a very interesting pattern emerges, for most of the population shows definite masochistic tendencies. It was to these that Professor Linton referred in discussing a distinctive part of the daily body ritual which is performed only by men. This part of the rite in-volves scraping and lacerating the surface of the face with a sharp instru-ment. Special women's rites are performed only four times during each lunar month, but what they lack in frequency is made up in barbarity. As part of this ceremony, women bake their heads in small ovens for about an hour. The theoretically interesting point is that what seems to be a preponderant-ly masochistic people have developed sadistic specialists.

The medicine men have an imposing temple, or latipso, in every com-munity of any size. The more elaborate ceremonies required to treat very sick patients can only be performed at this temple. These ceremonies involve not only the thaumaturge but a permanent group of vestal maidens who move sedately about the temple chambers in distinctive costume and headdress.

The latipso ceremonies are so harsh that it is phenomenal that a fair proportion of the really sick natives who enter the temple ever recover. Small children whose indoctrination is still incomplete have been known to resist attempts to take them to the temple because "that is where you go to die." Despite this fact, sick adults are not only willing but eager to undergo the protracted ritual purification, if they can afford to do so. No matter how ill the supplicant or how grave the emergency, the guardians of many temples will not admit a client if he cannot give a rich gift to the custodian. Even after one has gained admission and survived the ceremonies, the guardians will not permit the neophyte to leave until he makes still another gift.

The supplicant entering the temple is first stripped of all his or her clothes. In every-day life the Nacirema avoids exposure of his body and its natural functions. Bathing and excretory acts are performed only in the secrecy of the household shrine where they are ritualized as part of the body-rites. Pyschological shock results from the fact that body secrecy is suddenly lost upon entry into the latipso. A man, whose own wife has never seen him in an excretory act, suddenly finds himself naked and assisted by a vestal maiden while he performs his natural functions into a sacred vessel. This sort of ceremonial treatment is necessitated by the fact that the excreta are used by a diviner to ascertain the course and nature of the client's sickness. Female clients, on the other hand, find their naked bodies are subjected to the scrutiny, manipulation and prodding of the medicine men.

Few supplicants in the temple are well enough to do anything but lie on their hard beds. The daily ceremonies, like the rites of the holy-mouth-men, involve discomfort and torture. With ritual precision, the vestals awaken their miserable charges each dawn and roll them about on their beds of pain while performing ablutions, in the formal movements of which the maidens are highly trained. At other times they insert magic wands in the supplicant's mouth or force him to eat substances which are supposed to be healing. From time to time the medicine men come to their clients and jab magically treated needles into their flesh. The fact that these temple ceremonies may not cure, and may even kill the neophyte, in no way decreases the people's faith in the medicine men.

There remains one other kind of practitioner, known as a "listener." This witch-doctor has the power to exorcise the devils that lodge in the heads of people who have been bewitched. The Nacirema believe that parents bewitch their own children. Mothers are particularly suspected of putting a curse on children while teaching them the secret body rituals. The counter-magic of the witch-doctor is unusual in its lack of ritual. The patient simply tells the "listener" all his troubles and fears, beginning with the earliest difficulties he can remember. The memory displayed by the Nacirema in these exorcism sessions is truly remarkable. It is not uncommon for the patient to bemoan the rejection he felt upon being weaned as a babe, and a few individuals even see their troubles going back to the traumatic effects of their own birth.

In conclusion, mention must be made of certain practices which have their base in native esthetics but which depend upon the pervasive aversion to the natural body and its functions. There are ritual fasts to make fat people thin and ceremonial feasts to make thin people fat. Still other rites are used to make women's breasts larger if they are small, and smaller if they are large. General dissatisfaction with breast shape is symbolized in the fact that the ideal form is virtually outside the range of human variation. A few women afflicted with almost inhuman hypermammary development are so idolized that they make a handsome living by simply going from village to village and permitting the natives to stare at them for a fee.

Reference has already been made to the fact that excretory functions are ritualized, routinized, and relegated to secrecy. Natural reproductive functions are similarly distorted. Intercourse is taboo as a topic and scheduled as an act. Efforts are made to avoid pregnancy by the use of magical materials or by limiting intercourse to certain phases of the moon. Conception is actually very infrequent. When pregnant, women dress so as to hide their condition. Parturition takes place in secret, without friends or relatives to assist, and the majority of women do not nurse their infants.

Our review of the ritual life of the Nacirema has certainly shown them to be a magic-ridden people. It is hard to understand how they have managed to exist so long under the burdens which they have imposed upon themselves. But even such exotic customs as these take on real meaning when they are viewed with the insight provided by Malinowski when he wrote (1948:70):

> Looking from far and above, from our high places of safety in the developed civilization, it is easy to see all the crudity and irrelevance of magic. But without its power and guidance early man could not have mastered his practical difficulties as he has done, nor could man have advanced to the higher stages of civilization.

REFERENCES

Linton, R. The study of man. New York: D. Appleton-Century, 1936.
Malinowski, B. Magic, science, and religion. Glencoe, Ill.: The Free Press, 1948.
Murdock, P. Social structure. New York: Macmillan, 1949.

How would you feel about helping someone from this culture? When comparing this culture to your own, can you identify any similarities? Any differences?

At the *conclusion* of the group discussion, see Appendix II, p. 267.

Group

1. BROKEN SQUARES

This is a very popular activity whose original source is unknown. This exercise is helpful in investigating the concepts of problem solving, competition, cooperation, and nonverbal communication. It must be done in small groups of five participants with at least one observer per group. Each group is seated with the members facing one another around a flat working surface. The group is given a packet containing five sets of puzzle pieces—one set for each member. These packets are not to be opened until a signal is given and the game commences.

The individual objective is for each group member to construct in front of him or her a 6-inch square. The group objective is for five 6-inch squares to be constructed as rapidly as possible. As compiled, each envelope contains an insufficient number and selection of pieces to make a 6-inch square.

Specific rules for this game are:

1. No member may speak. You may not ask for puzzle pieces.
2. No member can signal, point, or otherwise nonverbally communicate for any reason.
3. You may not take puzzle pieces from another member, but you may freely give and receive pieces. Puzzle pieces must be given directly to a player; they may not be simply put in the middle for anyone to take.

The observer's task is to enforce the rules and watch the behavior of individuals.

This exercise elicits a high degree of involvement and interest from the participants. Discussion and sharing afterward may have to be directed by the group leader. Allow 1 hour for the exercise and discussion.

A description of how to prepare the packets and suggestions for the observer are in Appendix II, p. 267. *Caution:* Participants should *not* read Appendix II, or the impact of the game will be jeopardized! Only the organizer and observer should continue reading.

2. TINKER TOY EXERCISE

This exercise was adapted from Napier and Gershenfeld's "Tinker Toy Exercise," found in *Groups: Theory and Experience* (Boston: Houghton Mifflin, 1973). Needed: One or more cans of Tinker Toys. Participants: Randomly select 7 to 10 students to participate.

If there are verbal people in the class, put all of these folks in one group and the quiet folks in another group. Designate one observer for each group.

Have two groups work together in the same room. Put each group at a round table with no chairs. Make sure the two groups are in close proximity. Task: Give each group identical pieces of Tinker Toys. Allow students in each group 30 minutes to build a creation, using all pieces of the Tinker Toys. Members *cannot* talk to one another. *All* pieces must be used. Only toys should be on the table (remove boxes and directions).

The observers should familiarize themselves with the questions in Appendix II, p. 269, before beginning. *Caution:* Participants should *not* read Appendix II, or the impact of the game will be jeopardized! Only the organizer and observers should continue reading.

At the conclusion of the 30 minutes, each group is asked to present their creation. This explanation will include how and why the creation was designed. Members can talk about their feeling of being unable to communicate verbally. They also are asked to discuss the group process.

Observers will then be asked to discuss their findings from actually observing both groups in action.

3. SCHOLARSHIP AGREEMENT EXERCISE

Hames and Joseph have modified this exercise slightly, asking somewhat different discussion questions. The situations were developed by Lawrence B. Rosenfeld and published in *Human Interaction in the Small Group Setting* (Columbus, Ohio: Merrill, 1973).

Problem: To choose *one* of the following to receive a scholarship of $2000 per year to your school, renewable for 4 years as long as academic progress is satisfactory to the university.

Duane, 17, finished high school in 3 years because, he says, he "couldn't have stood another year of the b.s." His mother, a registered nurse, is a widow with two younger children. In spite of finishing a year early, Duane made a 3.0 in high school. University tests predict he is likely to earn a 2.6 in a science curriculum, 3.1 in nonscience. His mother is determined that he become a physician; Duane says his mind isn't made up. Because of the cost of baby-sitting her youngest child, his mother can provide almost nothing for his college education. Duane has had some emotional troubles; a psychiatrist recommends college because he feels Duane "needs an intellectual challenge."

Carla, 18, has very high recommendations from a small-town high school where she earned a 3.8 average. In her senior year she accepted an engagement ring from a local truck driver who wants her to get married at once and forget college. Your school predicts she is likely to earn a 2.6 in science and a 3.3 in nonscience. She wants to become a social worker "to help the poor in the big cities." Her pastor says she has a fine mind, but he predicts she will marry and drop out even if she starts college. Her parents are uneducated, industrious, and very poor.

Roy, 31, earned the Silver Star and lost his right hand in Vietnam. He earned a high school diploma in the Army. The university predicts a 2.0 in science and a 2.3 in nonscience for him. He is eligible for veterans' assistance, but his family needs his help to support a large brood of younger children. Roy wants to major in business, "to make enough money in my life so I can have a better life than my parents."

Melissa, 26, is a divorcee with a 7-year-old son. She made a 2.8 in high school, "because I goofed around," but tests predict a 2.9 in science at your school and a 3.6 in nonscience. She wants to become an English teacher, "probably in high school but in college if I'm lucky." She was a beauty queen at 18 and is still regarded as beautiful, but says she is bitter toward men and will never remarry. She receives no child support or family help toward caring for her son. Her present employer, a dress shop owner, gives her a good character reference but predicts she will marry again rather than finish college.

Sam, 19, was offered several football scholarships to southern colleges, but they were withdrawn when, after he finished high school, he injured his legs in an automobile accident. He can get around well but cannot compete in athletics. He made low high school grades, but entrance test scores for your school are good; he is predicted to average 2.5 in science or 3.0 in a nonscience curriculum. His father, a laborer, refuses to contribute to college for him. Now that he can no longer play football, Sam is determined to become a football coach, though he has been advised this may be difficult without a college playing record.

Divide the class into small groups of four to five people. Each group is asked to pretend they are the admissions committee of the university. You must make a decision as to which candidate should receive the scholarship and explain the rationale for your decision. Decide upon a leader. If no decision can be reached as to whom the scholarship is to be given, the leader must choose a candidate. You have 20 minutes to complete this exercise.

Assign one student to each group to observe the group process, noting who emerges as leader and how each of the members functions. Observers should discuss how a consensus was reached.

4. FISHBOWL

This exercise was developed by Patrick R. Penland and Sara F. Fine and can be found in *Group Dynamics and Individual Development* (New York: Dekker, 1974, p. 85).

In this task exercise, a fairly large group is divided into two groups. One group is assigned a task to accomplish and begins its group process. The other group sits in an outer circle and becomes observer to the acting group. This can be a most valuable experience in understanding group dynamics. Some of the issues for observation and discussion:

- What kinds of roles did individuals play? Can you name and describe them?
- What were the dominant processes of the total group?
- How would you describe the first part of the session as compared to the second?
- Were there implicit themes, a hidden agenda? Which of these were below the level of consciousness and not dealt with by the group?
- What kinds of behaviors seemed to be operating toward group movement?

- What forces were operating to hinder the task of the group?
- What kinds of participations were directed toward awareness of the personal experience within the group?
- Which members were moving toward task accomplishment and which toward open process?

Suggested topics for the group to work on:

1. Changing the present grading system of a course.
2. Changing present university policy regarding academic probation.
3. Playing a game such as Trivial Pursuit for a prize (winning team awarded candy or small amount of money collected beforehand; each student could donate a dime).

Threat

1. BUZZ GAME

This game is adapted from one you have probably played as a child. Its purpose is to demonstrate the effect that mild anxiety can have on functioning. The object of this game is to replace the number seven (7) or multiples of the number (7) by the word "buzz."

Directions

All group members are seated in a circle. One person starts the game by calling out the number one (1). The next person follows numerically, and so forth around the circle. Every time a number with a seven (7) in it, like seven (7), seventeen (17), or twenty-seven (27), or a number divisible by seven (7), like seven (7), fourteen (14), or twenty-eight (28), comes along, the person whose number it is does not say the number, but says "buzz." If anyone forgets to do so and says the number, the whole group must start over.

Discussion

After the game is over, consider these points for discussion: How did you feel as your turn approached, when it was your turn, when you successfully finished your turn, and when you missed? What was your reaction? How did the group as a whole react when someone missed?

2. THE ARM GAME

This game is adapted from Louis Bamonte in *Free to Live*, published in New York by Sadlier (1972). It helps the student identify biophysical, psychosocial, and cognitive manifestations of anxiety by engaging them in a process in which they will feel anxious. Students who are not feeling well or have known medical problems should *not* participate in this game.

Directions

1. Divide the classs into groups of four to eight.
2. Have each group stand in a row one behind the other. All participants must face the same direction.
3. When the leader gives the command to begin, all members must extend their arms to shoulder level with fingers pointing toward the walls, as in a wingspread.
4. The exercise is to be done in silence.
5. If one member of a group lowers his or her arms, the leader is to eliminate that group.
6. The last row of students to maintain the correct position wins.

Discussion

1. If you were anxious, describe your anxiety to other members of the class. What were some physical symptoms or behaviors you experienced? What kinds of thoughts were you thinking during the exercise? Were you afraid of what others in your group would say if you let them down?
2. What part does the concept of trust have in this activity? Relate trust to anxiety.
3. Identify threats you may have perceived.
4. Did you experience a conflict between what you would like to do (put arms down) and your responsibility to others (keep arms up)? What motivated you to keep your arms up as long as you did? Are you motivated in the same way when you have to do other things you do not particularly want to do?
5. How did the person who changed the positions of his or her arms first feel when the row was disqualified?
6. How did the other members of the group feel about the person who was responsible for their disqualification?
7. Did the task become more difficult because you could not see the faces of the person in your group? Do you think being toward the rear of the row made it different from being near the front or in the front?

3. ANXIETY AWARENESS

This exercise was designed by Professor Marylee Evans, College of Nursing, University of Rhode Island, to increase your self-awareness by generating thought in identifying daily anxious situations and usual strategies employed to reduce these anxieties.

Directions

1. The group leader writes the following on the board:

Threats	Reactions	Coping Mechanisms

2. Then each member is asked to share an experience that he or she finds threatening. These are listed in the first column. For example:

Threats
Studying for final exams; first date with someone new

3. Each member is then asked to discuss his or her reaction to this situation. Included in this answer are: (a) physical reactions, (b) emotional reactions, and (c) disturbances in ability to think clearly. For example:

Threats	Reactions
Studying for final exams	Butterflies, irritable, inability to recall information
First date with someone new	Increased perspiration, tell dorm mates about your date, images of how date will respond to you

4. After examining all the different reactions listed on the board, each one is asked to explain how their reactions are different or similar.

5. Following these explanations, each member is asked to discuss what his or her course of action usually is in an attempt to relieve this anxiety. Write these in the third column. For example:

Threats	Reactions	Coping Mechanisms
Studying for final exams	Butterflies; irritable; inability to recall information	Take frequent breaks; call friend to study with

Threats	Reactions	Coping Mechanisms
First date with someone new	Increased perspiration; tell others; wondering how date will respond to you	Wear extra deodorant, perfume; ask others for their opinion on how you look; putting anticipated negative responses out of your mind

6. How many and which kinds of coping mechanisms are successful in reducing anxiety for you?

4. A FARM NAMED ADAPTATION

This is an activity created by Jennifer Zimmerman Slattery, R.N., when she was a student at the University of Rhode Island. Its purpose is to help familiarize you with adaptive (defense) mechanisms and their role in reducing anxiety. Carefully read the following story and then answer the questions at the conclusion.

Life on the farm had been good. The old farmer was a kind man, and he loved and cared for all of his animals. The animals, in return, did all they could to make the farmer proud of them. Consequently, Adaptation Farm was envied as the most productive farm in all of Crisis County. At the big County Fair the previous year, Adaptation Farm had taken all the first prizes for farm animals. The plow horse was the strongest, the cow and goat gave the sweetest, richest milk, the pig was the fattest, the sheep had the softest wool, the rabbit had the most beautiful babies, and the chickens, ducks, and geese laid the largest double yolkers seen in those parts. Furthermore, the cat was the best mouser and the mouse the best hider. Even the owl, which lived in the rafters of the barn, was the wisest, and the old hunting dog was the most loyal. So everything had been peaceful and productive on the farm, and the animals were happy. Then there came a time of crisis. The farmer died.

All the animals were stunned. Shock and disbelief were common emotions within them all. Even the field mouse that lived under the farmhouse felt the loss, for there would no longer be crumbs and morsels dropped onto the floor from the old man's shaky hands. Perhaps the farmer's hunting dog had the most realistic perception of what had happened, for he too was old and would someday welcome the serenity of death. But, for now, it was up to him to organize the other confused and frightened animals. His first order was to instruct the animals to stay close to the farm. He told his friends that in order to decide the logical thing to do, they would all have to work together and pool their knowledge. A real threat existed that they might be broken up and placed on different farms. Presently, though, their thoughts seemed confused by their personal threats.

"Who will hitch me up to plow the fields?" complained the work horse.

"Who will milk us?" fretted the cow and goat. "We will become swollen and sore with soured milk."

"I'll never find enough to eat," moaned the already hungry pig.

"You think you have a problem," squawked the fowl. "Our eggs will pile high in their nests and go bad. Have you ever tried to climb up on a mound of rotten eggs every day to lay another—just to watch it rot!"

The sheep was quiet but thinking to himself, "My wool will be matted with burrs, and I'll die of the heat if I'm not sheared."

The cat was eyeing the mouse and rabbit hungrily, and they were both becoming afraid for their lives.

Even the owl was silently fretting, "I'll have no one intelligent to talk to. What shall I do?"

"Shut up, all of you," snapped the dog. "This self-pity is disgusting," he shouted, even though he himself already pined at the loss of his hunting companion. "We must think of the farm, not of ourselves. I want us all to meet here tomorrow morning. For now, don't go too far from the barnyard and for heaven's sake, cat, don't eat the mouse or rabbit. We must protect each and every member of this farm in order to think of a way to survive, understood?"

"Yes," mumbled the cat under his breath, as the glow from his eyes dulled. "I understand."

For the rest of the day, the gloom that had settled on the farm like a cold gray fog thickened, and one could have felt the mounting anxiety that crept into each animal's mind. The animals meandered without purpose around the barnyard, each falling slowly back into his own pit of self-pity.

The old dog spent the day in the farmhouse, lying at the foot of his master's empty chair, half dreaming of past good times and half trying to figure out what to do to keep the farm alive and whole. He relieved his anxiety by preoccupying himself with worries about each animal rather than his own. He was to become their leader in their fight for survival, and this kept his mind busy.

Later in the afternoon, the plow horse and the milk cow bumped into each other just outside the red barn, which sat to the left of the farmhouse. It was the only barn on the farm, so it was quite large because it housed all the animals at night and in bad weather.

"Horse, I don't know what's going to happen to me," complained the cow. "Who is going to milk me? I'll swell up and get sore. Oh my, will I get sore!"

"Stop complaining," snapped the horse. "This whole thing was your fault anyway. You must not have given enough milk for the farmer to drink."

"It was not my fault," sobbed the cow, even though she was ashamed of the fact that she had been low on production lately. "We cows have cycles, you know; that's nature," she further rationalized. "There was still plenty."

"I don't care what you say, it was still your fault," mumbled the horse as he started to walk away from the sobbing cow. He hadn't even heard what she had had to say; he just needed to find someone else to blame for this disaster.

The cow was then alone, upset, and wondering, "Maybe it was all my fault." Even then she could feel her insides begin to churn faster and faster in preparation for peak milk production. "Oh my," the cow complained to herself, "I'll bust for sure."

Just then the old goat came tearing across the barnyard and ran head on into the cow's already swollen belly.

"Ow," cried the cow. "What do you think you're doing, goat? Get out of here and leave me alone."

"Just having some fun, cow. Wanna fight?" challenged the goat as she lowered her worn and blunt horns for another charge.

"No!," screamed the cow. "Can't you see I'm in pain? My udder is already so sore I can hardly walk. Why don't you grow up, anyway? You're acting like a kid," the cow snapped as she painfully waddled toward the barn.

"Spoil sport," grumbled the goat as she scanned the barnyard for her next victim. Her gaze fixed on the sheep, who was grazing peacefully in the front pasture.

"Charge," she yelled as she raced across the lawn toward the unsuspecting sheep. "Here I come, ready or not," she screamed just before impact. At least she gave this victim some warning!

"Oof," grunted the sheep as he was hit broadside by the goat. "You're going to get it now!" retaliated the sheep, as he rose to his feet.

Then began the mock battle, with charges and retreats on both parts. Finally, the challenges became exaggerated with exhaustion to the point where they ceased in a heap of tired muscles and aching bones.

"That was fun," the sheep finally exclaimed. "Let's do it again tomorrow. I know how the farmer enjoys watching us play."

"But the farmer is dead," the puzzled goat stated.

"Tomorrow we'll have to play closer to the farmhouse so he can see better," the sheep went on, ignoring the goat's statement. "Yes, we'll have to do it again tomorrow," the sheep mumbled as he left the goat's side and wandered toward the watering trough.

The goat just remained lying in the green grass of the pasture, looking very puzzled.

Meanwhile, the horse had found some green grass to munch on the other side of the barn. He had been having a mental argument with himself as to who *was* to blame for the farmer's death. He mentally blamed every animal, save himself, for this disaster. Actually, everyone had been sloughing off a little on production, even himself. His mind reviewed each animal and what they had not done right in the last month, but his thoughts kept going back to what *he* had done wrong.

"Maybe I wasn't pulling hard enough at the plow and he had to push too much. No, the fowl haven't been producing enough eggs; that must have been what killed him. But he looked awfully tired last week after we tilled the potato field. No, it was that pesky mouse. He hasn't been cleaning himself well enough and the farmer caught some rare disease from him." This frustration and appeasement went on and on . . . .

The day dragged on and the mood remained gray. The ducks and geese were appeasing their inner guilt by laying more and larger eggs than they had ever laid before. The chickens were all laying more eggs, too, but they could not figure out why. The hen house was the only place on the farm that seemed alive with activity that afternoon. All the fowl were cackling and producing eggs like never before. Every laying box was filled with eggs, and each had either a chicken, duck, or goose sitting on each growing mound. In fact, soon there would be no room for more eggs and the fowl would begin laying on the floor.

The scene in the barn was so different. Everything was quiet. The mouse was determined to be impeccably clean. He seemed to be priding himself on a spotless coat, as he never had before. In the past he had been a normal mouse with a fairly clean coat and there was always a flea or two to keep him scratching. The rabbit too was quietly cleaning herself, as it appeared. However, she was being so diligent in her work, she was yanking out tufts of fur and making herself bleed from her overcleaned sores. She seemed to be enjoying this activity and did not realize what she was doing to herself. If this kept up, she would soon be bald and bloody!

The wise old owl was perched on a beam high in the rafters of the barn, observing the silent activity below. He could see the animals were all upset about something, but he could not remember what. This confused the owl, for how could he give his obviously needed advice if he could not remember what was upsetting them all? This further frustrated and upset the usually dependable owl. As he left his perch and gracefully flew out of the open loft door, he made a mental note to ask someone what was going on when he returned from his hunt.

The cat was too puzzled, as he lay in the warm sun of the windowsill. He recognized the fact that the farmer had died, but he could not figure out why everyone was so upset. He felt no sadness at the farmer's passing, and he could not seem to perceive what effect the old man's death could have on the future of the farm. He decided that he would not think about it any more and would just enjoy the last warming rays of the afternoon sun, snoozing on the windowsill. Maybe later he would chase the mouse around for exercise.

The sow spent most of the day searching for and eating food. Presently she was full because she had consumed what was left of her slop from the day before, plus the leftover chicken scratch, cow silus, and horse grain. So in the evening hours she had time to think of other things, which is rare for a pig. She was beginning to feel toward the other animals as she had for her litter the spring before. Her motherly instincts were strong, and she decided she would have to organize the farm animals if they were to survive. This leadership quality was not one of her normal assets, but she became desperate when she realized her food supply was now low. This urge to organize was strong; however, her energy levels were low, as is usual for a pig. "I'll think about it tomorrow," the pig thought as she drifted off to sleep.

That evening the animals slept. They were all exhausted from the day's worries and activities. The next morning the dog awoke in the same place he had spent the previous day, at the foot of his master's chair. He looked up sleepily hoping to see the old man sitting in the chair, but it was empty. His muscles and bones ached as he stretched the night's stiffness from his body. He sighed deeply as he remembered his sadness at his master's passing. He knew what he had to do. He must be strong to fulfill the role he had to, to lead the farm animals to health again. He slowly rose and strode toward the door. "This is going to be a long day," he said to himself as he stepped out into the morning sunshine.

1. Match each animal with the appropriate coping mechanism he or she used in the story. Explain why. Answers are in Appendix II, p. 270.

Dog _____	Compensation
Pig _____	Denial
Sheep _____	Dissociation
Goat _____	Introjection
Mouse _____	Projection
Chickens _____	Reaction Formation
Horse _____	Regression
Ducks and Geese _____	Repression
Cat _____	Sublimation
Owl _____	Undoing

2. These mechanisms are thought to function primarily to prevent or relieve anxiety. Was this true with each of the animals on the farm? How did these mechanisms affect their problem solving?

5. RESPONSES TO IMAGINED THREAT

Respond to the following excerpt from Edgar Allan Poe's "The Raven."

> Once upon a midnight dreary, while I pondered weak and weary,
> Over many a quaint and curious volume of forgotten lore—
> While I nodded, nearly napping, suddenly there came a tapping,
> As of some one gently rapping, rapping at my chamber door.
> "'T is some visitor," I muttered, "tapping at my chamber door—
> Only this and nothing more."

Close your eyes and think about what you have just read. Imagine that you are in a large old house alone on a dreary night. How do you feel? What in this poem do you identify as a threat? Do you personally respond to this threat with anxiety, fear, or stress?

6. PERCEPTION AND EMOTION

"The appearance of things changes according to the emotions. . . ." (Gibran, K., *The Treasured Writings of Kahlil Gibran*. Secaucus, N.J.: Castle Books, 1981).

Can you think of a time in your life when you let your emotions influence the way you perceived a situation and, hence, the way in which you responded to that situation?

Having learned to identify some of your reactions to threat, how have you managed to control them?

Helping

1. THE HELPING PROCESS

This is an exercise to develop your expertise in becoming an effective helper. Since you have read the chapter, you have some knowledge of the concepts presented and ideas about the role of helper and client. Recall the situation with Susan in the first example of Chapter 5.

Individual

Write responses to these questions:

- Is Susan asking for help?
- If so, what behaviors assist you in recognizing her need for help?
- How would you feel about helping Susan?
- As a professional helper, what would you like to know in order to assess the situation accurately?
- As a social helper, how would your method of helping differ from that of a professional helper?
- What do you think Susan's problem might be?
- How do you think Susan might respond to you?
- What might be your responses to her?

Group

Have one of your classmates or friends role play Susan and you be the helper. Try to help Susan while your class is quietly observing the process. It may be helpful for them to jot down notes of the interaction. At the end of your conversation with Susan, ask the class members for feedback about what they observed. Did you follow a process or the stages typical of relationships? In what ways did you intervene? How did Susan respond? Why were you—or were you not—helpful to Susan? Evaluate the relationship and discuss strengths and alternative ways of approaching Susan.

2. ROLE PLAYING

The purpose of this exercise is to help you to begin assuming a role as a professional helper. You are asked to reread the sections in the chapter that discuss the therapeutic climate and the role of the helper.

Now find someone to help.

Without informing the person of your aim, strike up a conversation with the intent of helping him or her if you can assess a need. Sit about 4 feet from the person, use direct eye contact, and be attentive. Make sure you dress appropriately and neatly for the situation. Observe the person for verbal and nonverbal responses. Make a mental note of these responses.

Repeat the above with either the same person or another. This time, however, when you talk with the person, avoid direct eye contact, sit in a slouched position, dress too casually or inappropriately for the situation, and frequently ask the person to repeat his or her verbal responses. Make a mental note of the person's verbal and nonverbal reaction.

Compare the results of each of your situations. What implications does this have to helping relationships, helpers, and clients? If you like, you might have an outside person observe your interactions in the two situations so that the observations will be more objective. If you do this, share your results with the other person at the conclusion.

3. HELPER OBSERVATIONS

This is an exercise designed to help you to begin to identify different types of helpers and how they assist people. Plan to observe at least three different types of helping professionals—doctors, nurses, teachers, social workers, pharmacists, etc. A suggestion is to observe the clients and helpers in a waiting room, classroom, or hospital.

Do these helpers try to establish trust? If so, how? If not, why not? What types of activities do these helpers engage in to facilitate the helping relationship? How do clients respond to this situation? Do clients share their problems with the helper? Consider the effectiveness of the relationship.

4. WILLOW IN THE WIND

This game was designed by Andrew Fluegelman. It is published in *More New Games!* . . . *and Playful Ideas from the New Games Foundation*, (Garden City, N.Y.: Doubleday, 1981, p. 67).

Imagine a warm summer night. Crickets are chirping, and graceful willows are swaying in a gentle, perfumed breeze. If we can imagine it, we can be there, with this New Games experience that cradles each of us in caring, supportive hands.

We form a small circle of about eight players standing shoulder to shoulder and facing the center of the circle with hands held at chest height, palms forward. Each of us should have one foot slightly behind the other for good balance. We've just transformed ourselves into a summer breeze, and now all we need is a volunteer to be the willow.

The willow stands in the center of the circle with feet together, arms crossed over the chest, and eyes closed. Keeping feet stationary and body straight but relaxed, the willow lets go, swaying from side to side, forward and back. Those of us in the circle support the willow with gentle pushes of our palms and provide summer-breeze sound effects. We should make sure that there are at least two people supporting the willow at all times and that our gentle breeze does not become a howling hurricane.

In turn, each of us gets to be the willow in the wind, swaying to and fro, caressed by the breeze. This is a trust game. The player who is the willow gets the opportunity to trust the other players completely, and those of us who are the breeze get to feel the trust the willow has placed in us.

5. LEADER-FOLLOWER TRUST WALK

This is taken from R. Napier and M. Gershenfeld, *Groups: Theory and Experience* (Boston: Houghton Mifflin, 1973).

The facilitator begins: "This exercise focuses on being a leader or a follower. Half of you will be blindfolded. Those who are not blindfolded will select a partner. This is a nonverbal exercise, so you may not speak to your partner to tell him or her who you are. Let's begin by counting off to two." (Participants count off "1, 2, 1, 2,"etc.) "Will all of the ones come to this side of the room? Here are handkerchiefs to use as blindfolds. Put them on and adjust them so that you cannot see." (The ones arrange their blindfolds and wait.)

Now the facilitator talks to the twos quietly so that the others cannot hear. "Each of you will select a partner from the group of ones. Stand beside the partner you choose so that we can determine who still needs a partner. Remember, you and your partner may not speak, but by all means try to develop a nonverbal language between you. You will be the leader. How can you help your partner experience the world? Can you enlarge your partner's world? Be aware of how you see your role; is it to protect your partner, to get your partner through safely? Is it to be with a minimum of effort on your part? Is it to be serious; is it to be fun? (Pause) Now select your partner.

"Explore your world—nonverbally, of course. I will see you back here in 15 minutes." (If this occurs in a building, 15 minutes is adequate time. If it is outdoors and time permits, allow longer. It is frequently a moving experience to see the partners develop their own signals, an increased sensitivity to each other, a trusting relationship.)

The facilitator alerts the group 2 minutes before time is up. If the setting is outdoors, the facilitator simply hopes that they will straggle back reasonably on time.

When they return, the "blind" remove their eye covers to see who their partners are. (This produces tension, anxiety, even fumbling, as the "leader" wonders if the follower will be disappointed when identities are revealed. There is also the anxiety of returning to the "real world," which does not encourage the closeness and trust some of the partners felt. Now the mood changes; the "uncovering" produces laughter, squeals of recognition, or surprise.)

The facilitator proceeds: "Would you share your feelings in the experience? What did you find out about yourself that was new? What did you find typical of yourself? How did you feel about your role—as a leader, or a follower?" (15 minutes)

"I am sure each of you wants to experience the other role. Will all of the twos come to this side of the room? Now it is your turn for the blindfolds. You know what to do."

The facilitator then talks to the ones as previously to the other group. Although they have been followers and know what they want their partners to experience, nevertheless it seems helpful to remind them, through the questions, of a variety of possible relations they may have with their partners in the leader role.

Once more, those not blindfolded select a partner and stand beside him or her. Frequently, the choosing partner will select the former partner to "repay" the partner for the interest he or she felt. For a variety of reasons, however, a person may prefer to select a new partner.

After selections are made, the exercise continues as in the first pairing. The groups return, see each other, share their feelings.

Sometimes the participants feel their reactions are significant and relatively private; they may only want to share with their partners. Sometimes participants are quite eager to share their new understanding of themselves with the whole group. If there is a group sharing, one of the questions the facilitator should ask is how it felt to be a leader and how it felt to be a follower. What was learned?

This exercise has usually been considered primarily an experience of trust; however, it is striking how often members report on their relations with authority. Students frequently note that it helps them understand their parents or gives them understanding of what kind of parents they would like to be. Men and women discuss their societal sex roles, in which a man is expected to be the leader, and their feelings when leadership roles are reversed. Some who usually see themselves as leaders are surprised at their reactions to being followers and gain a different perspective of the relationship; those who are usually followers give similar reports. Participants will also talk about clues they pick up from each other—being tired, bored, excited—that greatly influence the other person and the relationship; new insights are reported on complementary relationships.

As an aside, if a supply of handkerchiefs is difficult to attain, paper towels as they come from a dispenser and masking tape are equally effective as blindfolds.

Communication

1. OBSERVATION

This activity is designed to help you evaluate your observational skills and to practice giving clear and objective descriptions of other people. It should be done in small groups with approximately six students per group. Each group should choose a leader one class period prior to doing this exercise. It is the leader's responsibility to find a picture that depicts people engaging in several different activities. If possible, the picture should be in full color rather than black and white. The leader must not show this picture or discuss its contents with any group member.

When the group is ready to begin this exercise, one member is asked to leave the room. The leader then shows the remaining members the picture. Each member is allowed 60 seconds to look at the picture and, as completely as possible without taking notes, commit it to memory.

After one minute is over, the person who has not seen the picture is asked to come back into the room. At this time each member is asked to describe the picture to this person. After all members have had their turn, the member who originally did not view the picture is asked to describe what he or she thinks the picture looks like.

After this activity is completed, the leader will show the picture to the entire group. As a group, discuss the accuracy of your observations. Were you making value-free or value-laden observations? How well did you communicate to the person who did not see the picture? Did you observe the total picture or focus on certain aspects of the picture? Did you observe objects, persons, or both? Did certain activities taking place in the picture seem more important than others? Did you note colors used in the picture?

2. VERBAL COMMUNICATION

The purpose of this game is to assist you in perfecting your verbal communication skills. The specific aim is to encourage you to communicate in a clear, concise, and informative fashion.

This game is adapted from the telephone game you probably played as a child. You play by telling one person a story, having this person tell another person the same story, and so on. Eventually, the story gets to the last person, who reports to the group what he or she thinks the story is.

Since you now have a more advanced knowledge base regarding the theory of communication, your approach to this game will be somewhat different.

Directions

1. Divide into groups of six.
2. Choose a leader.

3. The leader must develop, in writing, a short story or message to be used for this game. It should contain a minimum of five sentences.
4. All members but the leader are asked to leave the room.
5. One member at a time returns to the room. The leader then tells this person the story.
6. This person in turn tells another group member his or her version of the story, and so on until each member has been told the story. (Written notes may not be used.)
7. The last member of the group tells the entire group his or her version of the story.
8. The leader reads the original story to the group.

Discussion

There are two perspectives from which to view this activity. The first is that of the sender. Did you concisely report the entire story? Were you influenced by distractors when attempting to give the message? Did you check for feedback? Did you ask specifically if the receiver understood your message? The second is that of the receiver. Were you influenced by distractors while trying to listen to the message? Did you ask the sender to repeat the message? Did you listen to the entire message or only part of it?

3. TRANSMISSION OF INFORMATION

The following exercise, whose source is unknown, is more sophisticated than exercise 2. Its purpose is to examine the differences between one- and two-way communication. Why not try your skill at both forms of communication?

Directions

1. Divide the class into groups of five, with an observer for each group.
2. One group will demonstrate one-way communication, while the other group will demonstrate two-way communication.

One-way Communication

In one-way communication, have the first person enter the room and read the story which follows once. After that person reads the story, ask the second person to enter and have the first person repeat the story. As the next person enters, have the second person repeat the story. Persons listening to the story may not ask questions. Continue this until the last person repeats the story to the observer.

Two-way Communication

In two-way communication, have the first person enter the room and read the story once. After that person reads the story, ask the second person to enter and have the first person repeat the story. In this type of communication, the second person may ask the first person questions about the story. Answer all questions. Once that person feels comfortable with the story, call in the next person and tell the story. Likewise, after that person is done, questions may be answered.

Observers

Record on observation sheet if a specific detail is reported (place a check mark) or if details are left out (place a zero). The observation sheet is in Appendix II, p 270. *Caution:* Only observers should read Appendix II or the game will be jeopardized!

The Story

A farmer in western Kansas put a tin roof on his barn. Then a small tornado blew the roof off, and when the farmer found it two counties away, it was twisted and mangled beyond repair.

A friend and lawyer advised the farmer that the Ford Motor Company would pay him a good price for the scrap tin, and the farmer decided he would ship the roof up to the company to see how much he could get for it. He crated it up in a very big wooden box and sent it off to Dearborn, Michigan—marking it plainly with his return address so that the Ford Company would know where to send the check.

Twelve weeks passed, and the farmer didn't hear from the Ford Company. Finally he was just on the verge of writing them to find out what was the matter, when he received a letter from them. It said, "We don't know what hit your car, mister, but we'll have it fixed for you by the 15th of next month."

4. NONVERBAL CUES

This is an exercise adapted from one developed by David W. Johnson (*Reaching out: Interpersonal effectiveness and self-actualization*, Englewood Cliffs, N.J.: Prentice-Hall, 1972, p. 107) that will help you recognize the difficulty in interpreting nonverbal cues. It is important for the helper to identify nonverbal cues and to recognize the necessity of collecting adequate information about the client before making a judgment about him or her.

Directions

1. Collect 10 pictures of people who seem to be expressing different types of emotion.

2. Give each picture a number, from 1 to 10.
3. Ask each group member to list the numbers 1 to 10 on a piece of paper.
4. Pass each picture around the group and ask members not to share their responses.
5. Have each member record *one* word that describes the emotion being depicted in the picture. Write the emotion for picture 1 on your paper. Do the same for 2 to 10.
6. Have each member share interpretations.

Discussion

Were some emotions easier to identify? For example, did most group members agree upon certain feelings for certain pictures? Were there some emotions that everyone disagreed upon? If so, why? How judgmental were you when making your decision about particular emotions? Were there certain nonverbal cues that made you decide upon a particular emotion, i.e., tears on a cheek, frowns, wrinkled brow, smiling face, pouty lips, or closed eyes?

5. SENSORY OBSERVATION

Although this exercise does not have to be completed in class, it is suggested that you record your observations and share them with your classmates. The purpose of this exercise is to help you utilize all your senses while making observations.

Directions

1. Work in small groups; approximately three students should be in each group. Choose a group leader.
2. The leader is responsible for finding two similar objects. Suggested items to use are two seashells, two potted plants, two rocks, two small ceramic figures, two similar but slightly different scents.
3. Before allowing the other two members to see the objects, blindfold one member, thus preventing him or her from using the sense of sight to make observations.
4. Give each member five minutes to examine the objects.
5. Ask each member to write down his or her findings before members talk about this experience with one another.

Discussion

Did the person who was blindfolded utilize his or her other senses—smell, sound, taste, and touch—more often? Were the findings made by each member similar or different? Did the person who was blindfolded make less value-laden comments, i.e., avoiding terms like "pretty," "beautiful," or "expensive"? When asked to examine, did the person who was not blindfolded utilize mainly the sense of sight? When you shared this information with your entire class, did you discover any consistent findings?

6. MAKE YOUR OWN MODEL

Adler & Towne (*Looking Out/Looking In*, 3rd ed. New York: Holt, Rinehart and Winston, 1981, p. 27) developed the following exercise:

Check your understanding of the communication model by applying it to your own life.

1. In a group of three, share two important messages you intend to express within the next week.
2. For each message, describe:
   a. The idea you want to send and the various ways you could encode it.
   b. Channels by which you could send it.
   c. Problems your receiver might have in decoding it.
   d. Possible differences between your environment and that of the receiver, and how those differences might make it difficult to understand your full message.
   e. Likely sources of external, physical, and psychological noise that might make it difficult for you to phrase your message clearly or for your receiver to understand it.
   f. Ways you can make sure your receiver uses feedback to verify an accurate understanding of the message.

7. RECOGNIZING YOUR EMOTIONS

Adler & Towne (*Looking Out/Looking In*, 3rd ed. New York: Holt, Rinehart and Winston, 1981, p. 97) developed the following exercise:

Keep a 3-day record of your feelings. You can do this by spending a few minutes each evening recalling what emotions you felt during the day, what other people were involved, and the circumstances in which the emotion occurred.

At the end of the 3-day period you can understand the role emotions play in your communication by answering the following questions:

1. How did you recognize the emotions you experienced: through nonverbal behaviors, cognitive processes, and/or verbal expression?
2. Did you have any difficulty deciding which emotion you were feeling?
3. What emotions do you experience most often? Are there any emotions

that you did not experience as much as you would have expected?

4. In what circumstances do you/do you not express the feelings you experience? What factors influence your decision to share or not share your feelings? The type of emotion? The person(s) involved? The situation (time, place)? The subject that the emotion involves (money, sex, etc.)?

5. What are the consequences of the type of communicating you just described in step 4? Are you satisfied with these consequences? If not, what can you do to become more satisfied?

Hames and Joseph propose a sixth question:

6. Does "getting in touch" with your feelings facilitate your understanding of the events that have occurred during this 3-day period?

8. PROCESS RECORDING

The process recording is an analytical report of a helper's interaction with a client. It is an exact written report of the conversation between the helper and client. It provides an opportunity for the helper to:

1. Accurately focus on the client's needs.
2. Explore the reasons for a response and the possible effects it might have had on the communication process.
3. Become more aware of his or her own strengths and weaknesses when communicating in a therapeutic fashion.
4. Use this awareness as a base for assimilating new knowledge and skills in relation to therapeutic communication and use of oneself to help others.

Directions

1. Choose a situation in which you assume the role of a helper with a client. Although this recording may be done with a friend, it is important that the portion of the situation you choose to record is one in which he or she is actively attempting to discuss feelings about a problem.
2. Describe briefly the client and the situation under which you were helping him or her.
3. List your communication goals.
4. Write the process recording like the script of a play. *Note the example given in Chapter 8.* This script portion should be written under the column labeled *Interaction.*
5. Write exactly what the client says and your response. Use quotation marks.

6. In parentheses indicate all the nonverbal cues you noted, i.e., tone of voice, mannerisms such as finger tapping, distractors.
7. After recording your interaction, use the column labled *Techniques* to name each of those responses that were therapeutic and non-therapeutic.
8. In the *Analysis* column, critique each of your responses. Include why you felt they were helpful or not helpful to the client. Where appropriate, suggest responses that might have been more therapeutic.
9. Summarize the interaction in paragraph form at the end. Read the recording thoroughly and write down your thoughts concerning the interaction. Analyze it from different points of view where possible. Ask such questions as: With what parts was I satisfied and with what parts was I dissatisfied? Why? Is there a different approach? Does this show habitual patterns of responding on my part? On the part of the client? Include a discussion of your utilization of the elements of communication.

Note

It is beneficial to write the recording shortly after the interaction if possible. If not, jot down that which is pertinent and will help you to recall major points when you do write it down later that day. Write down exact words used. It is not expected that you will always respond in a therapeutic fashion. It is more important that you begin to recognize when and why you use non-therapeutic techniques. Interpretation of what is going on occurs all the time and often very unconsciously. It is helpful to us to make this as conscious a matter as possible and to distinguish in our recording between an observed fact and our interpretation of that fact. Conscious analysis and interpretation help us to respond to feelings people are trying to express and not merely to the words they may be using.

9. ROLE PLAYING

Practice is the only way to become proficient at utilizing therapeutic communication skills. Thus, role playing becomes a very important factor when you are attempting to perfect your ability to use these skills. Although at first you may feel uncomfortable with role playing because it is not real, you must remember the advantages of being able to make mistakes in the classroom where no real clients will be affected.

If you have videotape equipment or a tape recorder available, it will be especially beneficial to record this exercise. By using this equipment you will have instant feedback that will be invaluable to you in critically analyzing your performance as a helper. If this equipment is not available, role play with other classmates observing and recording your performance. Also talk to the persson who assumed the role of client during the role-playing exercise. Did this person find your interventions therapeutic? Did this person feel comfortable, that you cared about him or her as a person? Both the observer's and the client's perspective can be very enlightening.

The following situations designed by Hames and Joesph are suggestions for role-playing exercises. Each situation gives you some information about what has happened and what emotion the client is feeling. If you are assuming the role of client, try to convey some emotion when talking to the helper. Remember, these are only parts of situations; you are expected to role play and create more of a story from this given situation. It is also hoped that you will devise your own situations and continue to practice role playing.

Situation 1

You are a sophomore in college. After taking your midterm in biology, you have become very anxious and upset. The exam was much more difficult than you anticipated. You feel sure that you have failed.

Situation 2

You have just accepted a fraternity pin from Tom, whom you have been dating since you were a junior in high school. Since you are now a freshman in college, you have mixed feelings about making this commitment to Tom. You think that you would like to start dating others but you do not want to hurt Tom's feelings. You feel trapped.

Situation 3

Your parents have just cut off your funds for college because they have learned you are living with John. You are angry that they are not more considerate of you as a person. You feel that they do not respect your judgment about people. Also, you feel that your parents see this as a moral issue and fail to recognize that you are a person of very high principles.

Situation 4

Your children are 10 and 12 years old. You have decided to return to college to finish the degree you began 15 years ago. You are excited and enthusiastically awaiting the beginning of school. Unexpectedly, you learn that you are pregnant—much to your dismay! You are 33 years old, and you feel that this baby will ruin your plans to go back to school. You are shocked and very depressed.

Situation 5

Your father was a football hero in college. He was responsible for scoring the winning touchdown in several important games. Even today at age 46, he is very athletic, playing tennis and jogging almost daily. You have just been delegated to the second string of the football team and spend most of the games warming the bench. Although your father has done nothing to make you feel he is disappointed in your ability, you are upset about not being as athletic as your dad.

Situation 6

Mrs. Henderson, a 75-year-old widow, has been raising her 12-year-old grandson since he was 2. She is a deeply religious woman, believing that God will take care of the two of them. Lately she has not been feeling well, and she is worried about what will happen to her grandson if she is seriously ill.

Situation 7

Adam, aged 6, and Donald, aged 4, have been playing together every day all summer. Lately Adam has been complaining to his mother that he does not want to play with Donald every day. He says that Donald is babyish and wants his own way all the time.

Situation 8

You have just made a midlife career change to go back to college and become a nurse. You like school, and you are doing well. Last night you were offered a job as director of a social work agency in upstate New York. The starting salary is $30,000, and they want you very much. Although you really want to be a nurse, you know that your salary will not reach $30,000 for several years. You feel frustrated; you want to continue with school but feel you are not being practical.

Situation 9

Your 10-year-old son has been caught stealing from a local Woolworth's. You are shocked and disappointed in him. You also are feeling guilty because you've had such a busy schedule lately and have not been able to spend much time with him.

Situation 10

Your father, aged 53, has been diagnosed as having terminal cancer. You feel the need to go back home and be with him. However, that would mean dropping out of school for a semester, which would add an extra financial burden on your mother later. *The decision is up to you;* your mother has not tried to influence you.

Situation 11

Your mother called you last night to tell you that your dad and she are getting a divorce. He has found someone else. Your mother begged you never to see him again, feeling that he has deserted all of you. You have always loved your dad, and you *want* to see him, but you don't want to hurt your mother.

10. COMMUNICATION QUIZ

The following quiz designed by Hames and Joseph will help familiarize you with the therapeutic and nontherapeutic techniques of communication. There are two sections of this quiz. Part I will help you identify therapeutic techniques and Part II will help you recognize the effects of nontherapeutic communications upon the client. The answers for both parts can be found in Appendix II, p. 272.

Part I

Match the following:

_____ 1. *Helper:* I'm not sure I understand. Could you tell me more?

_____ 2. *Client:* I feel so sad.
Helper: Sad?

_____ 3. *Client:* Should I take French this semester?
Helper: Yes, then you'll have your language requirement filled.

_____ 4. *Client:* I'm afraid I'm flunking English. I will not pass the final exam.
Helper: You'll pass—after all, you haven't failed anything yet.

_____ 5. *Client:* I feel awful; I'm so dizzy.
Helper: Did you feel this way all day or did this just happen?

_____ 6. *Client:* My dad is really sick. I hated to leave him this morning.
Helper: Don't worry so much—you can always call to see how he his.

_____ 7. *Helper:* Tell me about your visit with the doctor.
Client: Well, I really feel good about it . . .

_____ 8. *Client:* I'm really afraid . . . I don't think I'll be able to cope.
Helper: Why do you feel scared?

_____ 9. *Helper:* Tell me about your study habits before we talk about your grade.

A. Broad opening statement
B. Offering self
C. Asking why questions
D. Minimizing the client's feelings
E. Interrupting
F. Changing subject
G. Probing
H. False reassurance
I. Placing event in time sequence
J. Silence
K. Giving advice
L. Trite expression
M. Seeking clarification
N. Summarizing
O. Reflection

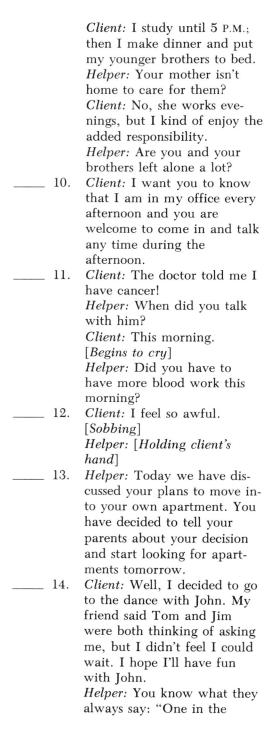

Client: I study until 5 P.M.; then I make dinner and put my younger brothers to bed.

Helper: Your mother isn't home to care for them?

Client: No, she works evenings, but I kind of enjoy the added responsibility.

Helper: Are you and your brothers left alone a lot?

_____ 10. *Client:* I want you to know that I am in my office every afternoon and you are welcome to come in and talk any time during the afternoon.

_____ 11. *Client:* The doctor told me I have cancer!

Helper: When did you talk with him?

Client: This morning. [*Begins to cry*]

Helper: Did you have to have more blood work this morning?

_____ 12. *Client:* I feel so awful. [*Sobbing*]

Helper: [*Holding client's hand*]

_____ 13. *Helper:* Today we have discussed your plans to move into your own apartment. You have decided to tell your parents about your decision and start looking for apartments tomorrow.

_____ 14. *Client:* Well, I decided to go to the dance with John. My friend said Tom and Jim were both thinking of asking me, but I didn't feel I could wait. I hope I'll have fun with John.

Helper: You know what they always say: "One in the

hand, is worth two in the
bush."

_____ 15.   *Client:* On Tuesday, I'm going to . . .
Helper: To start classes.
Client: Yes, I can hardly
wait. But I'm kind of . . .
Helper: Well, it is exciting,
isn't it?

Part II

Match the following:

_____ 1. Asking questions—probing
_____ 2. Minimizing the client's
           feelings
_____ 3. False reassurance
_____ 4. Changing the subject
_____ 5. Giving advice
_____ 6. Trite expressions
_____ 7. Jumping to conclusions
_____ 8. Inappropriate use of facts
_____ 9. Interruption
_____ 10. Prolonged silence

A. Remarks that tell the
    client how to feel. They
    close the door to the
    communication process.
B. Creates client depend-
    ency and imposes helper's
    value system upon the
    client.
C. Offering factual informa-
    tion to client without
    regarding client's feelings
    about the situation.
D. Implies that the client's
    feelings are not unusual
    and not important.
E. Breaks the flow of the
    conversation. Client is
    unable to express a com-
    plete thought or feeling.
F. Makes the client feel un-
    sure and puts him or her
    on the defensive.
G. Solving problems
    prematurely. The client
    fails to investigate all
    alternatives.
H. Minimizes the
    significance of the client's
    feelings. Conveys a lack
    of truly understanding or
    being interested in the
    client. Promises outcomes

that may not happen.

I. Allow client to drift from topic being discussed.

J. Takes the focus of the conversation away from the client, therefore blocks what the client is attempting to discuss.

11. ACTIVE LISTENING

Adler and Towne *(Looking Out/Looking In, 3rd ed. New York: Holt, Rinehart and Winston, 1981, pp. 227–228)* developed the following exercise:

1. Find a partner; then move to a place where you can talk comfortably. Designate one person as A and the other as B.
2. Find a subject on which you and your partner apparently disagree—a current events topic, a philosophical or moral issue, or perhaps simply a matter of personal taste.
3. A begins by making a statement on the subject. B's job is then to paraphrase the idea back, beginning by saying something like "What I hear you saying is . . . " It is very important that in this step B feeds back only what she or he heard A say without adding any judgment or interpretation. B's job is simply to *understand* here, and doing so in no way should signify agreement or disagreement with A's remarks.
4. A then responds by telling B whether or not his or her response was accurate. If there was some misunderstanding, A should make the correction and B should feed back his or her new understanding of the statement. Continue this process until you are both sure that B understands A's statement.
5. Now it is B's turn to respond to A's statement, and for A to help the process of understanding by correcting B.
6. Continue this process until each partner is satisfied that he or she has explained him- or herself fully and has been understood by the other person.
7. Now discuss the following questions:
    a. When you were a listener, how accurate was your first understanding of the speaker's statements?
    b. How did your understanding of the speaker's position change after you used active listening?
    c. Did you find that the gap between your position and that of your partner narrowed as a result of your both using active listening?
    d. How did you feel at the end of your conversation? How does this feeling compare to your usual emotional state after discussing controversial issues with others?
    e. How might your life change if you used active listening at home? At work? With friends?

12. DEAF DONALD

"Deaf Donald" is from *A Light in the Attic; Poems and Drawings* by Shel Silverstein. Copyright © 1981 by Snake Eye Music, Inc. (By permission of Harper & Row, Publishers, Inc.) Discuss the poem. Consider now communication skills can be either effective or ineffective. Discuss the importance of nonverbal skills.

Deaf Donald met Talkie Sue

 But 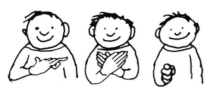 was all he could do.

And Sue said, "Donald, I sure do like you."

But  was all he could do.

And Sue asked Donald, "Do you like me too?"

But 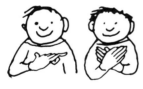 was all he could do.

"Good-bye then, Donald, I'm leaving you."

But 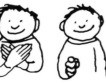 was all he did do.

And she left forever so she never knew

That  means I love you.

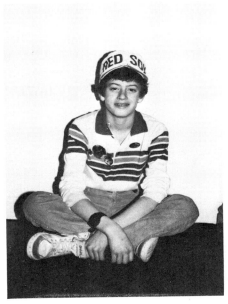
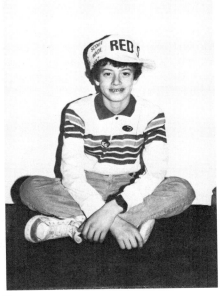

A   B

13. OBSERVATIONAL QUIZ

You have 30 seconds to do the following exercise. Please time yourself. Note carefully photo A and photo B. List the differences in photo B. After you have completed this, turn to Appendix II, p. 272, for a list of the differences. (Photo credits to Peggy Haggerty.)

Learning

1. SIMULATED TEACHING-LEARNING

This group activity designed by Hames and Joseph will provide you with an enjoyable teaching-learning experience upon which you can base discussion. Prior to doing this, you should spend time thinking about something you could teach someone. You should have a fair degree of knowledge and experience with the subject. Bring needed materials with you to class.

To start, divide into pairs or into groups of three, if you would like to have the benefit of an observer. (Note to observer: Guidelines for Observers are included in Appendix II, p. 273. Only observers should refer to this prior to the exercise.) The two participating people should designate one person to be the "teacher," and the other the "learner." Within a designated period of time, it is your task to "teach" and "learn" effectively. At the conclusion of this activity, participants and observers should share their experiences and feelings with one another and with the rest of the group. Relate your discussion to your readings. For specific questions to consider, refer to the Guidelines for Observers. Note: An alternative to this exercise is to have the learner blindfolded or handicapped in some other way.

2. MY LEARNING STYLE

Keep a detailed record of study habits for 4 days. Evaluate how you learn best. Do you look at the whole situation and then examine the parts? Do you look at each part before examining the whole? Do you learn only by reading words, or do you utilize other sensory cues? Do you read an assigned chapter before class or days and weeks after a related lecture? The following is an example of how you might keep track of your record. Be prepared to discuss your learning styles in class.

TOPIC: MUSIC 101 INTRODUCTION TO CLASSICAL MUSIC

Date	Assignment	Learning Process	Style Used
2/1/84	Must know about Mozart and his music for exam next week	Read in text about Mozart's life, the early years, 1–12	Visual—only looked at one portion of his life
2/2/84	Same assignment	Listened to Mozart's works written at age 12. Continued to read in text using highlighter which helps to visualize important areas	Visual—color helpful Hearing—listened to music. Still looking at one portion of Mozart's life
2/3/84	Same assignment	Listened to later works. Finished reading about Mozart's life	Visual Hearing Continue to look at one portion
2/4/84		Participated in play *Amadeus*, about Mozart's life	More physical as well as mental involvement Put whole life in perspective

3. HIDDEN FIGURES TEST

This is adapted from the well known Group Embedded Figures Test (GEFT), originally developed by Philip Oltman, Evelyn Raskin, and Herman Wilkins. It is a test of your ability to distinguish parts from the whole. Time yourself. See how long it takes you to locate each of the lettered figures A to E in the numbered patterns below. There is only one figure in each pattern and this figure is always right side up and the same size as shown. How did you arrive at the answers? What strategies did you use? Was it frustrating?

The answers are in Appendix II, p. 273.

PART I

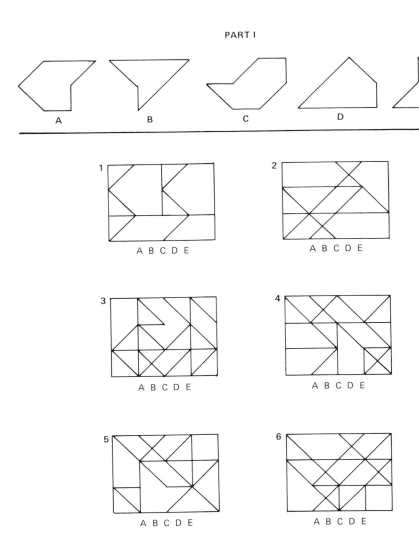

PART II

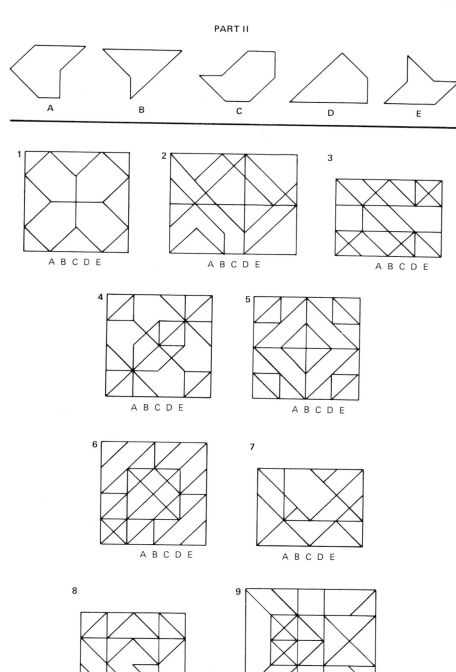

PART III

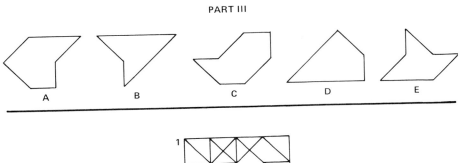

A   B   C   D   E

1

A B C D E

2

A B C D E

3

A B C D E

4

A B C D E

5

A B C D E

6

A B C D E

7

A B C D E

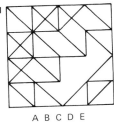
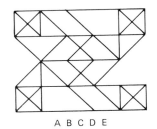
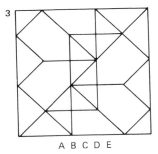
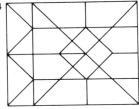
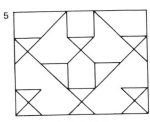
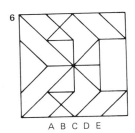

Problem Management

1. INDIVIDUAL DECISION MAKING

Problem Analysis

Select a problem that you have had today, i.e., what to eat for breakfast or which movie to go to tonight. Using the steps of problem solving, review your decision making.

1. Identify your need. Compare how things were with how you desired or needed things to be. Note the difference.

   _____

2. State the problem.

   _____

3. Compose an objective stating the behavior you want to demonstrate.

   _____

   The necessary components are:
   Subject _____
   Behavioral verb _____
   Conditions _____
   Criterion for measurement _____

4. State each alternate solution you considered. Under each alternative list:

The Positive Factors	The Negative Factors

   On a scale of 1 to 5, rank each alternative according to its probability and ease of outcome:
   (Least Likely)   1   2   3   4   5   (Most Likely)

5. State the method (intervention) by which the objective will be accomplished.

   _____

   The necessary components are:
   Subject _____
   Recipient _____
   Object _____
   Time _____
   Briefly justify your choice.

   _____

6. Describe how you implemented the chosen alternative; include responses to your action.

_____

_____

_____

7. Evaluate the outcome. Was it successful or not? _____
   List:

Things That Went Well	Things That Did Not Go Well

Make a statement regarding present need for termination, continuation, or modification.

_____

_____

2. WRECKED ON THE MOON

This is an exercise in individual and group decision making, developed by Jay Hall. Working by yourself, place the items listed in the order of importance as instructed. Prepare a justification for your decision based upon systematic problem solving. Now, as a group, try to rank order the items in such a way that each member can at least partially agree upon the decision. Reach agreements by discussing alternative opinions, not by arguing or simply having someone "give in." If you are working with a group greater than six to eight, it is possible to subdivide into several small groups and then compare the consensus of each. The correct answers are included in Appendix II, p. 276.

Instructions

You are a member of a space crew originally scheduled to rendezvous with a mother ship on the lighted surface of the moon. Due to mechanical difficulties, however, your ship was forced to land at a spot some 200 miles from the rendezvous point. During reentry and landing, much of the equipment aboard was damaged and, since survival depends on reaching the mother ship, the most critical items available must be chosen for the 200-mile trip. Below are listed the 15 items left intact and undamaged after landing. Your task is to rank order them in terms of their importance for your crew in allowing them to reach the rendezvous point. Place the number _1_ by the most important item, the number *2* by the second most important, and so on through number *15*, the least important.

Your Answer		Group Answer	Correct Answer
	Box of matches		
	Food concentrate		
	Fifty feet of nylon rope		
	Parachute silk		
	Portable heating unit		
	Two .45-caliber pistols		
	One case dehydrated Pet milk		
	Two 100-lb tanks of oxygen		
	Stellar map (of the moon's constellation)		
	Life raft		
	Magnetic compass		
	Five gallons of water		
	Signal flares		
	First aid kit containing injection needles		
	Solar-powered FM receiver-transmitter		

At the conclusion of this exercise, it may be helpful to have the group discuss the method by which it solved the problem. Why was this method used? Were members able to participate and share their ideas easily? If not, why? Did a leader emerge? What kind of behaviors impeded or facilitated the group process? Did you have to change your original rank ordering? If so, do you feel that you just "gave in" or that you understood why you were changing your original priorities? Did the group develop a "spirit" or "sense" of survival? Did everyone willingly participate?

3. BRAINSTORMING

This exercise, adapted from Napier and Gershenfeld (*Groups: Theory* and experience. Boston: Houghton Mifflin, 1973) by Hames and Joseph, is to help you begin examining how the problem-solving process works.

Brainstorming is a technique used to help generate ideas that will eventually help solve problems. This activity can be lots of fun, as it tends to stimulate your creativity. Follow these simple directions:

As a group (in class) identify a problem you need to solve. You can make up your own problem, or you can try one of the problems suggested:

- Changing the structure of a present course;
- Changing the grading system on campus;
- Changing the present political structure;
- Changing a particular policy or rule on campus.

Now follow a few simple rules (have one member read to class).

1. All ideas are to be respected—no criticism allowed.
2. Be open—explore the wildest of ideas—there are no boundaries.
3. Generate as many ideas as possible.
4. Persons may give one idea at a time; you must allow all members to participate.

Now, as a large group, decide upon a problem. Then divide into smaller groups. Assign someone to be a recorder in each group. Allow 15 minutes for the groups to generate ideas. Return to the larger group and share brainstorming ideas.

Discussion

Did one group generate more interesting ideas? If yes, why?

Did you come up with a different quality of ideas as you allowed yourself to fantasize?

Did you have a tendency to be critical of suggestions? If yes, what happened? In this early phase of problem solving is "criticism" important?

4. COMMON TARGET GAME

This exercise is designed to show how the human problem-solving process needs to be based on a sound theory and systematic approach to problem management.

Directions

Your instructor will divide the class into groups of five, with each group assigning a game coordinator.

Instructions to Game Players

The members of each group are not allowed to communicate with one another in any way. You must be seated back-to-back so that you cannot observe other members in the group.

The game coordinator will announce to each group a number between zero and 40. Each member has been given a set of cards numbered one to ten. At the coordinator's command, each member of the group will be instructed to raise a card displaying the amount he or she wishes to contribute to help the group reach its target number. If a game player wishes to contribute no points, simply raise your hand.

The coordinator will quickly total all the cards displayed and announce the total to the group. The coordinator *will not* tell who has contributed what amounts, simply the total. The group will repeat this process until the target number has been achieved. Once it is achieved, a new target number will be announced. The objective of the exercise is to minimize the number of trials the group takes to achieve each of several target numbers.

COMMON TARGET COORDINATOR RECORDING FORM

Target	Number of Trials	Target	Number of Trials
19	_____	9	_____
3	_____	18	_____
31	_____	35	_____
13	_____	24	_____
25	_____	34	_____
6	_____	29	_____
20	_____	17	_____
12	_____	30	_____
28	_____		
36	_____		**STOP**
26	_____	38	_____
37	_____	33	_____
39	_____	8	_____
21	_____	4	_____
	STOP	32	_____
14	_____	11	_____
15	_____	27	_____
16	_____	23	_____
1	_____	22	_____
2	_____	10	_____
7	_____	5	_____
		40	_____
			STOP
			Total Trials ____

Instructions to Game Coordinators

1. Allow NO COMMUNICATION among members.
2. Accurately total all cards.
3. DO NOT MAKE ANY COMMENTS THROUGHOUT THE EXERCISE, simply announce the total shown!

4. Give plenty of time for each member to think about what he or she wants to contribute.
5. Use the commands CARDS UP and CARDS DOWN after each attempt.
6. Continue on the same target number until it is achieved.
7. After your first set of targets, ask the group to stop and communicate quietly about the process.
8. Resume the game with the second set of targets and stop at the appropriate place.
9. THERE IS *NO COMMUNICATION* BETWEEN GAME COORDINATOR AND GAME PLAYERS!

Discussion

Have each group discuss feelings evoked while playing this game. What was frustrating? Did you feel anger? At whom? Were your communication sessions productive? If you were going to play again, how would you change your strategy?

Appendix II

Answers and Special Instructions for Activities

Answers and special instructions to games and exercises are in this section. The contents of this appendix should *not* be read by participants.

Adaptation

LETTER AND ASSESSMENT

This exercise is found on page 216.

Mode		Stimuli	Response	Behavior
Biophysical	(f)	Car won't start	Circulation affected by temperature—vasoconstriction	Anticipated: numbness, frostbite—absence of circulation, fingers and toes appear black
	(c)	Temperature outside—subnormal	Decreased blood supply to extremities ∴ untoward behaviors (noted in behavior column)	Actual: tingling noted in hands and feet Pain in hands Feet freezing Exhaustion

Mode	Stimuli	Interpretation	Response
	(c) "Healthy"	Circulatory system will be able to withstand this extra taxation	Continues to shiver, rubs hands together, keeps moving Anticipated: collapse
Psychosocial	(f) Car won't start Looking forward to teaching (c) 35-year-old teacher (c) Today was supposed to be an "early day" (c) Planned to go shopping (c) Repairman (c) Began day with cheerful mood	Frustration	Actual: Swearing: "Wickford is damn ugly" Believes repairman is happy car won't start Telephoning proper place to get car fixed States sense of humor lost
Cognitive	(f) Car won't start (c) College teacher (c) Knows how to get repair help (c) Focus is on immediate situation only	Intellectual immobility—obviously capable person but has not carefully prepared for cold weather	Actual: improperly clothed for weather—no warm boots, not wearing warm gloves Left notes for lecture in car

The above interaction depicts one moment in time. Since you know virtually nothing about the teacher, it is unlikely that you will have identified any residual stimuli. Note that the focal stimulus—car that will not start—remains constant in all three modes or domains. Stimuli do not have to be biophysical in nature to evoke a biophysical response. In turn, psychosocial or cognitive stimuli also could induce a biophysical response, or a biophysical stimulus could produce a psychosocial or cognitive behavior. It is interesting to note that carefully assessing these stimuli adds a richness to the assessment, which would be lost if the helper decided to investigate one mode solely.

Culture

ON THE VARIOUS MEANINGS OF WORDS

This exercise is found on page 220.

9	1.	Blade
10	2.	Busted
7	3.	Bread
1	4.	Boss
3	5.	Copout
8	6.	Freeze
5	7.	Choice
2	8.	Heavy
4	9.	Checkout
6	10.	Come outa your act

NACIREMA

This exercise is found on page 220. What does Nacirema spelled backwards mean? Try rereading the cultural description!

Group

BROKEN SQUARES

This exercise is found on page 224.

Directions for Preparing the Packet

You need a set of five envelopes containing pieces of cardboard that have been cut in different patterns, and that, when properly arranged with pieces from some of the other four envelopes, will form five squares of equal size. One set should be provided for each five-member group. To prepare a set, cut out five cardboard squares of equal size, approximately six by six inches. Place the squares in a row and mark them penciling the letters a, b, c, etc., lightly so they can be erased later. Use accompanying diagrams as a guide.

   The lines should be drawn so that when cut out, all pieces marked "a" will be of exactly the same size, the pieces marked "c" will be of exactly the same size, and the pieces marked "f" will be of exactly the same size. By using multiples of three inches, several combinations will be possible that will enable participants to form one or two squares, but only one combination is possible that will form five squares six by six inches.

After drawing the lines on the six-by-six inch squares and labeling them with the lowercase letters, cut each square as marked to make the parts of the puzzle.

Mark each of the five envelopes A, B, C, D, and E. Distribute the cardboard pieces in the five envelopes as follows:

- Envelope A has pieces i, h, e.
- Envelope B has pieces a, a, a, c.
- Envelope C has pieces a, j.
- Envelope D has pieces d, f.
- Envelope E has pieces g, b, f, c.

Erase the penciled lowercase letter from each piece and write on it, instead, its appropriate envelope letter. This will make it easy to return the pieces to the proper envelope for later use when a group has completed the task. Remember to make one complete set for each group of five participants. It may be helpful to use different construction paper for each set.

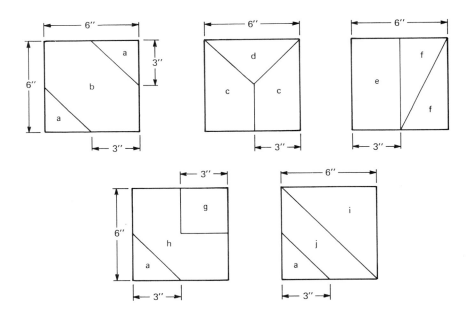

Suggestions for the Observer

As observer you are responsible for making sure that the participants play the squares game according to the directions. Since you do not have an emotional involvement in the game, you are in a unique position to more objectively observe the participants' responses to each other and the task.

Specifically, watch for and be prepared to share those behaviors that relate to frustration, cooperation, competitiveness, and nonverbal communication. How do members handle individual and group problem solving in this environment? What kind of behaviors impede or facilitate the group process? What nonverbal reactions do members exhibit as they work? Which members seemed willing to give up their pieces—to destroy their squares to help others? Did some members withdraw from playing the game once their square was formed? Did a leader emerge? Did one person figure out how to solve the problem and willingly share this information with others? Did individuals and groups seem to compete with each other?

TINKER TOY

This exercise is on page 225.

Suggestions for Observers

1. How do individuals in the group arrange themselves around the table (randomly, friendship subgroups, etc.)?
2. At the end of the task, how has this initial ordering been changed? In front of whom is the final product? Why? Has this person the most skill? Is he or she the best organizer? Is he or she the most popular? Doe he or she have the most power?
3. To which people in the group was most of the nonverbal communication directed? Were others encouraged to share their ideas in some manner?
4. Did members "jump" on one of the first ideas communicated, or did they seek to explore alternatives? Did all the participants really understand what they were building when they started, and did they seem to agree with the idea?
5. How were tasks distributed during the work period? Was there any organization of labor, or did individuals just do what came naturally?
6. Were particular roles (facilitating and inhibiting) identified within the group?
7. What did individuals who were obviously not directly involved in the decisions or perceived as resource people do to compensate for feelings of noninvolvement, inpotency, or even inadequacy in this particular group?
8. Did particular behaviors by individuals (no names are necessary, but it is helpful if the group can accept direct feedback) create defensive responses in other members? Responses should be specific about the action and reaction parts to this question.

9. How did the group respond to the pressure of time and to the pressure of the group working next to them? Did they relate to the group next to them?
10. What norms developed as the group began to work together? Did these change as the task progressed?
11. What types of leadership styles were exhibited within the group, and what impact did these have upon the developing group climate?

Other observations relating to membership, subgrouping patterns, tension release, and reward and punishment in the group may be explored. It also is important to observe how the two groups use each other as outlets for their own feelings.

Threat

A FARM NAMED ADAPTATION

This exercise is found on p. 231.

Dog	Sublimation
Pig	Introjection
Sheep	Denial
Goat	Regression
Mouse	Reaction formation
Chickens	Compensation
Horse	Projection
Ducks and Geese	Undoing
Cat	Dissociation
Owl	Repression

Communication

TRANSMISSION OF INFORMATION

This exercise is found on p. 241.

Observation Sheet

Listed in the first column are the 20 details of the story. As Person 1 repeats the story to Person 2, note the mistakes in Person 1's version by writing the wrong words or phrases in the proper row and column. To help you with scoring, use a check mark for details correctly reported and a zero for the details left out. Repeat this procedure for the remainder of the participants.

Item	Original Story	Version 1	Version 2	Version 3	Version 4	Version 5
1	Farmer					
2	Western Kansas					
3	Tin roof on his barn					
4	Small tornado					
5	Two counties away					
6	Twisted and mangled					
7	Friend and lawyer					
8	Ford Motor Company					
9	Good price					
10	Ship the roof					
11	How much he could get					
12	Very big wooden box					
13	Dearborn, Mich.					
14	Return address					
15	Send the check					
16	12 weeks passed					
17	Verge of writing					
18	Received a letter					
19	What hit your car					
20	15th of next month					

COMMUNICATION QUIZ

Part I

This quiz is found on p. 249.

1. M	6. D	11. F
2. O	7. A	12. J
3. K	8. C	13. N
4. H	9. G	14. L
5. I	10. B	15. E

COMMUNICATION QUIZ

Part II

This quiz is found on p. 251.

1. F	6. A
2. D	7. G
3. H	8. C
4. J	9. E
5. B	10. I

OBSERVATIONAL QUIZ

This exercise is found on p. 254.

The following differences exist in photo B:

1. Hat moved
2. Collar buttoned
3. Large buttons removed
4. Watch on different arm
5. Shirt sleeves down
6. Arms in first picture, left over right; second picture, right over left.

Learning

SIMULATED TEACHING-LEARNING

This exercise is found on p. 254.

Guidelines for Observers

While you are watching the participants engage in the teaching-learning activity, consider the following. Prepare to discuss them.

1. The attitude of the teacher toward the subject being taught and toward the learner: does he or she appear knowledgeable and sincere about the subject? Does he or she have positive regard for the learner?
2. Can you see evidence of the teacher's utilizing all four steps of the teaching process: assessment, design, interaction, and evaluation?
3. What style of teaching does the teacher seem to be most comfortable with? What frustrates him or her? How effective is he or she? Offer suggestions.
4. Can you see evidence in the learner of any of the following: readiness, motivation, understanding of what is being taught, supportive opportunities, and opportunities for success and evaluation? If so, describe. If not, dicuss how these could have helped learning in this situation.

HIDDEN FIGURES TEST

This exercise is found on p. 256.

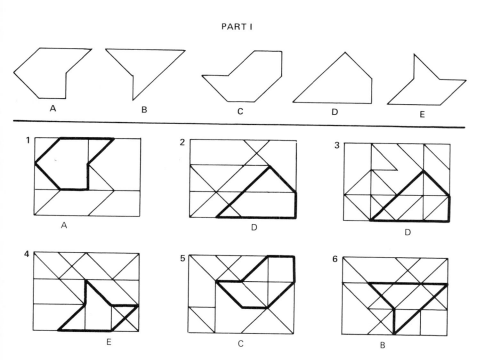

PART I

PART II

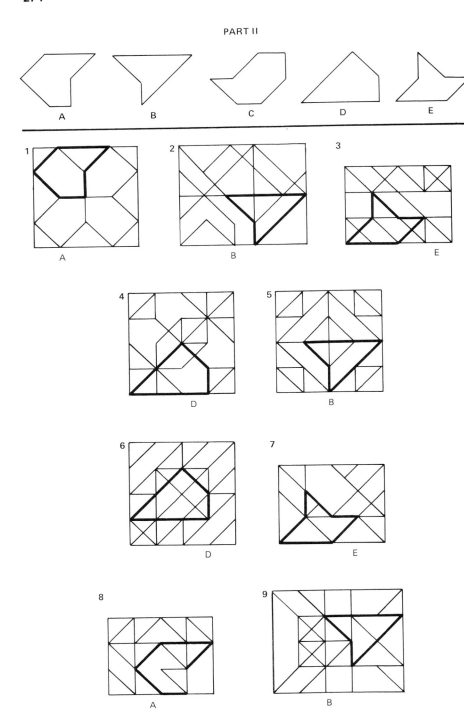

PART III

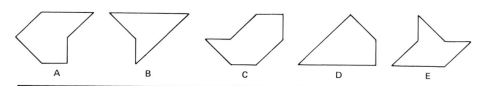

A   B   C   D   E

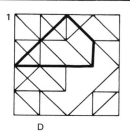

D

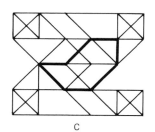

C

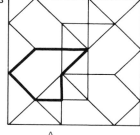

A

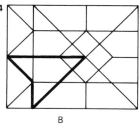

B

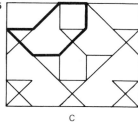

C

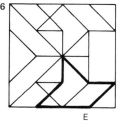

E

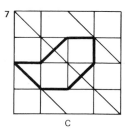

C

Problem Management

WRECKED ON THE MOON

This exercise is found on p. 260.

The following listing is the correct rank ordering of items needed for survival:

Answer		Rationale
15	Box of matches	No O_2 on moon
4	Food concentrate	Efficient means of supplying energy for what may be days of traveling
6	Fifty feet of nylon rope	Useful in scaling cliffs and tying injured together
8	Parachute silk	Protection from sun's rays
13	Portable heating unit	Not needed on lighted side where overheating, not cold, is a problem
11	Two .45-caliber pistols	Possible means of self-protection or self-propulsion device
12	One case dehydrated Pet milk	Bulkier duplication of food concentrate and utilizes water supply
1	Two 100-pound tanks of oxygen	Most pressing survival need for even the shortest amount of time
3	Stellar map (of moon's constellations)	Primary means of navigation to locate own position as well as directions to mother ship
9	Life raft	CO_2 bottle used in raft can be used for propulsion. May be used to carry supplies or injured
14	Magnetic compass	No magnetic field
2	Five gallons of water	Replacement of liquid loss; basic survival need
10	Signal flares	Only good on dark side; may serve as distress signal or propulsion device
7	First-aid kit containing injection needles	Needles will fix aperture in space suits; may contain valuable medicines
5	Solar-powered FM receiver-transmitter	Increases communication ability to mother ship; may allow you to send a distress signal

Appendix III

Statements on a Patient's Bill of Rights

1. The patient has the right to considerate and respectful care.
2. The patient has the right to obtain from his physician complete current information concerning his diagnosis, treatment, and prognosis in terms the patient can be reasonably expected to understand. When it is not medically advisable to give such information to the patient, the information should be made available to an appropriate person in his behalf. He has the right to know, by name, the physician responsible for coordinating his care.
3. The patient has the right to receive from his physician information necessary to give informed consent prior to the start of any procedure and/or treatment. Except in emergencies, such information for informed consent should include, but not necessarily be limited to, the specific procedure and/or treatment, the medically significant risks involved, and the probable duration of incapacitation. Where medically significant alternatives for care or treatment exist, or when the patient requests information concerning medical alternatives, the patient has the right to such information. The patient also has the right to know the name of the person responsible for the procedure and/or treatment.
4. The patient has the right to refuse treatment to the extent permitted by law, and to be informed of the medical consequences of his action.
5. The patient has the right to every consideration of his privacy con-

Affirmed by the Board of Trustees, American Hospital Association, November 17, 1972.

cerning his own medical-care program. Case discussion, consultation, examination, and treatment are confidential and should be conducted discreetly. Those not directly involved in his care must have the permission of the patient to be present.

6. The patient has the right to expect that all communications and records pertaining to his care should be treated as confidential.

7. The patient has the right to expect that within its capacity a hospital must make reasonable response to the request of a patient for services. The hospital must provide evaluation, service, and/or referral as indicated by the urgency of the case. When medically permissible a patient may be transferred to another facility only after he has received complete information and explanation concerning the needs for and alternatives to such a transfer. The institution to which the patient is to be transferred must first have accepted the patient for transfer.

8. The patient has the right to obtain information as to any relationship of his hospital to other health-care and educational institutions insofar as his care is concerned. The patient has the right to obtain information as to the existence of any professional relationships among individuals, by name, who are treating him.

9. The patient has the right to be advised if the hospital proposed to engage in or perform human experimentation affecting his care or treatment. The patient has the right to refuse to participate in such research projects.

10. The patient has the right to expect reasonable continuity of care. He has the right to know in advance what appointment times and physicians are available and where. The patient has the right to expect that the hospital will provide a mechanism whereby he is informed by his physician or a delegate of the physician of the patient's continuing health-care requirements following discharge.

11. The patient has the right to examine and receive an explanation of his bill regardless of source of payment.

12. The patient has the right to know what hospital rules and regulations apply to his conduct as a patient.

Appendix IV

The American Nurses' Association Code of Ethics (1976)

1. The nurse provides services with respect for human dignity and the uniqueness of the client unrestricted by considerations of social or economic status, personal attributes, or the nature of health problems.
2. The nurse safeguards the client's right to privacy by judiciously protecting information of a confidential nature.
3. The nurse acts to safeguard the client and the public when health care and safety are affected by the incompetent, unethical, or illegal practice of any person.
4. The nurse assumes responsibility and accountability for individual nursing judgments and actions.
5. The nurse maintains competence in nursing.
6. The nurse exercises informed judgment and uses individual competence and qualifications as criteria in seeking consultation, accepting responsibilities and delegating nursing activities to others.
7. The nurse participates in activities that contribute to the ongoing development of the profession's body of knowledge.
8. The nurse participates in the profession's efforts to implement and improve standards of nursing.

From the American Nurses' Association *Code for Nurses with Interpretive Statements,* Kansas City, Mo., The Association, 1976.

9. The nurse participates in the profession's efforts to establish and maintain conditions of employment conducive to high quality nursing care.

10. The nurse participates in the profession's effort to protect the public from misinformation and misrepresentation and to maintain the integrity of nursing.

11. The nurse collaborates with members of the health profession and other citizens in promoting community and national efforts to meet the health needs of the public.

Index